What the experts are saying about *KidShape* . . .

"[*KidShape* will] get your family motivated to a healthier, thinner future. *KidShape* gives the tools to prevent not only obesity, but other serious medical conditions as well, including diabetes and high blood pressure."

—RESA LEVETAN, MD; Professor and Chief of Endocrinology, Diabetes, and Metabolism; Drexel University College of Medicine; author of *Day by Day Diabetes*

"Dr. Neufeld has designed a program that has proven effective [in helping overweight children]. This book is a practical do-it-yourself, how-to guide to help you implement a similar program for your own family."

—HELENA W. RODBARD, MD, FACP, MACE

"KidShape reflects the lessons we have all learned together to fight obesity. I have watched this program as patients and their families came, hungry for an awareness of the distress they feel and for education about nutrition."

—CHRIS LANDON, MD, FAAP, FCCP; Founder of the Landon Pediatric Foundation; Director of Pediatrics and the Pediatric Diagnostic Center, Ventura County Medical Center, Ventura, California

"If you have children who are overweight, if you know children who are overweight, or if you are simply concerned about stopping the epidemic of obesity and related illness that is threatening our children today, then you must read this book. Dr. Neufeld provides the means to restore and preserve our children's health."

—DONALD BERGMAN, MD; President, American Association of Clinical Endocrinologists; Clinical Associate Professor of Medicine, Mount Sinai School of Medicine, New York, New York

"Any parent with an overweight child should read *KidShape* to learn how to become informed consumers of healthy foods in a marketplace filled with confusion. Here are commonsense solutions that work. I highly recommend *KidShape*."

—DAVID HEBER, MD, PhD; Professor of Medicine and Director, UCLA Center for Human Nutrition; author of *The L.A. Shape Diet*

"Dr. Neufeld gives parents the tools and direction to improve the health of everyone in the family."

—YANK COBLE JR., MD, MACE, MACP; Past President of the American Association of Clinical Endocrinologists; Past President of the American Society of Internal Medicine

You can talk online with other concerned parents about KidShape. For day-to-day support, join fellow readers on the KidShape message board on iVillage.com at www.ivillage.com/kidshape. (If you don't have Internet access at home, you can sign on at your local library.) Here you can find inspiration, answers, and encouragement from families who are making this program part of their lives.

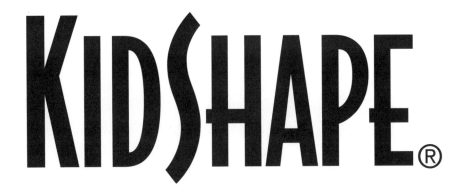

KIDSHAPE®

A PRACTICAL PRESCRIPTION
FOR RAISING HEALTHY,
FIT CHILDREN

NAOMI NEUFELD, MD, FACE

WITH PETE NELSON

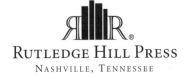

RUTLEDGE HILL PRESS
NASHVILLE, TENNESSEE

A Division of Thomas Nelson Publishers
Since 1798

www.thomasnelson.com

Published by Rutledge Hill Press, a Division of Thomas Nelson, Inc., P.O. Box 141000, Nashville, Tennessee 37214.

KidShape® Registered U.S. Patent and Trademark Office.

Many of the figures, tables, discussion questions, and worksheets in this book have been adapted from *The KidShape Student Workbook, The KidShape Parent Workbook,* and *The KidShape Program Manual,* copyright © 2003, 2002, 2001, 1999, 1998, 1997 by the KidShape Foundation. This material has been adapted with the permission of the KidShape Foundation.

The information in this book is for general knowledge only. Before beginning this or any other diet and exercise program, consult with your child's health care provider, as well as your own health care provider. Seek prompt medical care for any specific medical problem or concern.

Food and exercise illustrations by Nina Kidd.

Library of Congress Cataloging-in-Publication Data

Neufeld, Naomi, 1947–
    KidShape : a practical prescription for raising healthy, fit children / Naomi Neufeld with Pete Nelson.
        p. cm.
    Includes bibliographical references and index.
    ISBN 1-4016-0141-3 (pbk.)
    1. Children—Nutrition. 2. Obesity in children—Prevention. I. Nelson, Pete. II. Title.
RJ206.N397 2004
618.92'39805—dc22   2004000423

First and foremost, to my husband,
Tim, whose love and support helped me to
realize my goals at a time when KidShape was
just a good idea.

To my daughters, Pam and Kathy, who
continue to be my joy and inspiration.

To my parents, Dilip and Maya Das,
who encouraged me to fulfill my dream
of becoming a physician.

Finally, to all the families who struggle
with weight problems every day. I hope
this book will lead the way to a healthier
and happier way to live.

Contents

Acknowledgments

An endeavor that touches so many lives is necessarily the result of the labors of many dedicated and passionately committed people. I have been extremely lucky to work with Christiane Wert Rivard, MPH, RD, the program director of KidShape for the past eight years. She is smart, savvy, and tireless—she even runs marathons for fun—and is an incredible role model. KidShape owes its vitality to the efforts of several people, including Beth Braun, PhD; Mandy Graves, MPH, RD; Mary Jarrett; and Peter Sartini. And of course, we at KidShape could not survive our own day-to-day marathons without the dedication and energy of our office staff: Brenda Quintero, Yamille Acosta, and José Morales.

The KidShape program is taught by a staff of highly skilled and creative professionals who are dedicated to improving the lives of the families with whom they work. It is for these families, who have come to us, believed in us, and from whom we learn every day, that I have the greatest thanks

I am grateful for the encouragement of professional colleagues, including Chris Landon, MD, of the Pediatric Diagnostic Center in Ventura, California, and David Heber, MD, a fellow endocrinologist and the director of the Center for Human Nutrition at UCLA. Both have extended support to KidShape during its growing pains. Elisa Nicholas, MD, medical director of the Children's Clinic in Long Beach, California, has been a staunch supporter and a strong advocate for KidShape in the public health arena. Juditha Pascual, director of Children's Nutrition Services for the County of Los Angeles, has been an ally, an advocate, and a friend to KidShape since the beginning.

Of course, there would be no book were it not for the encouragement, confidence, and persistence of my agent Todd Shuster of Zachary Shuster Harmsworth. I am grateful to the wonderful people at Rutledge Hill Press whose vision, generosity, and compassion have brought this book to reality. I thank Jennifer Greenstein and Pete Nelson for countless hours and great skill in helping me to get these ideas out clearly. Finally, I am thankful to Teresa Sanchez, whose diligence and dedication, as well as her calm and organized nature, allowed me to work on this book and maintain my clinical practice.

Introduction and Overview

Congratulations.

You've bought this book (or perhaps you're still browsing in the bookstore) because you think your child is overweight. Perhaps you *know* your child is overweight, but you don't know what caused it, what to do about it, or where to turn. Perhaps you've already tried different weight loss regimens, and either they didn't work or the child has regained the lost weight. Maybe you have considered a new fad diet, but you don't know what's right or safe for kids. Or maybe you haven't addressed the weight problem because you're afraid of embarrassing or emotionally damaging your child.

I say congratulations—because you've already taken the first step. You are doing something about it, and you're asking all the right questions. That can be the hardest thing to do. Many good, loving parents are in denial about their child's weight, or feel guilty or responsible for it and can't address it. Relax— you've come to the right place.

As the former director of pediatric endocrinology at Cedars-Sinai Medical Center in Los Angeles and current director of the KidShape family-based pediatric weight management program, I've spent the last 20 years addressing all the questions just mentioned. I've seen countless parents enter my office, overweight child in tow, everyone apprehensive and anxious, and I've seen them a few months later, hopeful and glad, knowing they're on the right track.

I want you to know three things:

→ You are not alone.

→ You are not to blame.

→ You have great reasons to hope.

You may already know that you're not alone. Of late the news media has emphasized the fact that America is suffering not just from a weight problem but also from a serious obesity epidemic, adults and children alike. It's not just you or your family: Americans in general are too fat. You don't need me to tell you that, because you can look around in any restaurant or store and count the people you see who are overweight.

In this book we'll examine more closely the nature of the problem, because it's important for you to understand what you're up against. If you feel that it's a complicated situation that isn't easy to understand, you're right. It is. It also can seem completely overwhelming. Our world and the food we eat have changed in many ways to make us prone to weight gain.

But there's plenty you can do about it, and most of it is fairly simple.

That's the great irony, and also the good news. Obesity and overweight are the number one health problem facing Americans today, but we know how to treat it: diet and exercise. Doctors have understood for some time that the key to improving our health is making a lifelong change in our activity levels and the ways we eat. We also know that the earlier your family begins with healthy habits, the easier it will be.

How do you get started, and how do you learn to continue these good habits?

That's what I've been working on for the past two decades. Beginning in 1984, in my pediatric endocrinology practice I began to see increasing numbers of overweight children—many as young as five years old. As the number of overweight children referred to me continued to increase, it quickly became evident that pediatricians often did not know how to handle the problem, and that standard approaches to fitness don't work with children. I repeatedly watched children's eyes glaze over during discussions of diet and exercise. As the crisis grew, I knew I had to find a better way to confront this unhealthy development. I wanted something that would be effective and permanent, that could be applied to all kinds of families in all kinds of situations—to families like yours.

In 1986 my colleagues and I set up a family-based weight management program for children as young as six years old. The child and parent attended the eight-week program together and received a structured education in nutrition and exercise. We called the program KidShape, and it was the first program to use the power of the entire family—the family table—to bring about permanent change. We'd seen the principles of family therapy applied to other behavioral problems, but no one had ever tried it with diet—would an educational system based on the family work to help overweight kids lose weight?

The answer is yes. Over the years, working with families rich and poor, we've helped more than 10,000 children lose weight by learning how to make healthy choices about eating and activity. (The figures below show the change in average daily fat/sweet consumption, average weekly hours of physical activity,

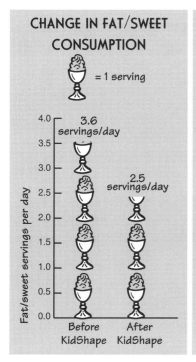

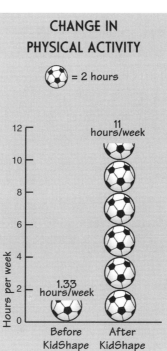

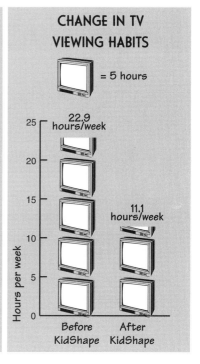

and average weekly hours of television viewing for KidShape participants.) Of those 10,000 kids, more than 8,000 kept the weight off—an astounding success rate for weight loss programs. We've also discovered that most of the *parents* who participate in this program also lose weight and dramatically improve their own fitness, vitality, mood, and stress levels, and help vanquish many weight-related health problems. Today KidShape offers programs throughout California, as well as in Texas, New Mexico, and Pennsylvania, and it is recognized by state and private health insurance carriers.

The good news is that the principles of the KidShape program can work for you in your own home, without your being part of the outside program. When families lose weight together, they reinforce each other in ways that personal trainers or aerobics instructors cannot. It works for kids because kids model themselves after their parents; it works for parents because parents work hard to keep the promises they make to their children. The reasons for overeating often begin to disappear when communication channels open. Where eating and exercise are concerned, knowledge is power, and knowledge is teachable, even for small children. The skills you need to apply that knowledge to your daily lives are teachable too. And where eating and exercise are concerned, there's no better place to teach, practice, and reinforce healthy habits than in your own home.

> *"We are more physically active and depend on TV less."*
>
> —KidShape parent

All that is needed is your time. You will meet in your home, as a family, for a workshop about once a week, though you will work at your own speed. Each workshop will involve reading, discussion, questions and answers, and fun activities—it will take about two hours, but you can split it into several meetings if needed. You will listen to your children, and give them positive reinforcement. You will make a commitment to your children to exercise with them for at least 30 minutes three times a week, and more if you can manage it. You will sign a contract, keep food and activity logs, and help your kids complete homework assignments. You may complete a workshop in a day or two, or you may want to stretch it out across several weeks. In the end, you will lose weight, and feel better, and feel closer as a family. I will guide you as you apply the methods and practices tried and tested over the last 15 years in our clinics.

For all the fat jokes and the comic actors wearing fat suits in movies, there's nothing funny about being overweight. Your overweight children are at serious risk for life-limiting and life-threatening health problems.

By buying this book, you've taken the best first step you could have taken. I would advise reading the whole book before beginning the program, though you may want to begin right away. Realize that you will be making subtle life-long changes in the way you eat and exercise without immediate gratification, but filled with the promise of lasting gratification. You will also be having a lot of fun along the way.

Let's get started.

Chapter 1

How We Got Here

When Goldilocks broke into the house of the three bears, at the table she found three bowls of porridge: one too hot, one too cold, and one just right—three bowls ready and waiting for a family of bears preparing to sit down and eat together.

Imagine that.

If Goldilocks were breaking and entering today, she'd probably find a bowl in the microwave with a note taped to it saying, "Baby Bear, Had to work late—here's your dinner. Have fun at soccer practice. Love, Mama Bear." Papa Bear would be in front of the television eating a pizza that he picked up on his way home, and he'd be finished by the time a stressed-out Mama Bear got home, tired from work, to eat her dinner cold while standing at the kitchen sink. If Goldilocks were to hang around, she might see Baby Bear finally burst through the door hours later to say the soccer team ate at McDonald's after the game, before heading to his room to play Nintendo.

You're Not to Blame!

Some readers may remember a time, not that long ago, when families broke bread together, everyone eating the same food at the same time in the same place, two meals a day and sometimes three, if the kids lived close enough to school to come home for lunch. The food was prepared by a stay-at-home mom, serving as *de facto* family nutritionist, chief cook, and bottle washer. She planned the weekly menu and did all the marketing, setting steaming bowls of provisions before her family. You can still see families like that on sitcoms from the 1950s and 1960s, *Leave It To Beaver* or *Father Knows Best*. As they ate, everybody took turns reporting on their days at school, at work, at play, at home, or discussed who was going to take whom to the prom, or which little brother stole which big brother's baseball mitt.

> *"KidShape understands kids and talks to them in a language that they understand without offending them."*
>
> —KidShape parent

Today the family meal seems like the exception to the rule. For thousands of years, the shared meal was the place where family lore was passed down and familial bonds were established and reinforced. Now that may only happen on special occasions, birthdays, or holidays. Whether we like it or not, the world has changed dramatically. How many times in the last week did you eat on the go? Eat standing up? Eat while driving in your car? Eat out? Nibble on junk food? Eat in front of the television, talking to other family members only during the commercials? Eat alone? Zap your food in the microwave because you were in too much of a hurry to prepare it any other way? Go to the supermarket without a weekly menu plan, buying instead what tempted you?

We have, of course, had "junk" foods since the 1950s, back when McDonald's kept track of the number of hamburgers they'd sold, posting the figure proudly outside their franchises. Today fast-food franchises seem to be on every corner—even in many other countries. It's not surprising that Great Britain, China, and Japan, where U.S. fast-food chains have proliferated, are now seeing more weight-related health problems than ever before.

Everything today is geared toward convenience. Look around your neighborhood and you'll see that convenience stores and mini-marts (which rarely have more than a token basket or two of fresh fruits or vegetables) have replaced most neighborhood grocery stores. Even the corner gas station has remodeled into a convenience store or mini-mart.

The result is lots of relatively cheap, easily available, highly flavorful foods and drinks of dubious nutritional value. Those foods themselves have changed in many ways, beginning in the 1970s with the introduction of high-calorie high-fructose corn syrup to replace sucrose or dextrose. High-fructose corn syrup, six times sweeter than cane sugar, enhanced the shelf life of processed foods, points out Greg Critser in *Fat Land*. It was more economical than other sweeteners and lowered prices, but also added calories to our diets. The other additive finding its way into our food in the 1970s was palm oil from Malaysia, a cheap high-calorie vegetable oil with the chemical properties of beef fat and more highly saturated than hog lard. At least one study, reported in the *Annals of Nutrition and Metabolism*, has linked it to problems with blood sugar (by increasing insulin resistance).

These cheaper ingredients allowed suppliers of fast or processed foods to increase portion sizes. Thus a 200-calorie serving of McDonald's fries in 1960 ballooned to a 610-calorie super-size serving. A convenience store 64-ounce soda is now five times the size—and five times the calories—of a regular can of soda.

You can see why we are eating far more fat and sugar than ever before, and an average of 200 more calories a day than 25 years ago. And the results are clear: Today 35 percent of American adults (59 million people) are overweight, according to the *International Journal of Obesity and Related Metabolic Disorders,* and another 26 percent are 30 or more pounds overweight. An astounding 9 million people are what is called morbidly obese, 100 pounds or more overweight.

The Age of Sedentary Living

It might not matter so much if we were all burning more calories a day than we did in 1977, but we're not. The reverse is true: These days we tend to be less active, not more active.

Don't feel guilty—all your best intentions are at war with the way you are made. The human body developed to survive lean times, famine, drought, and food shortages, by creating a complex mechanism to store fat for times of need. The body stocks up on spare calories during times of abundance. The problem is that your body failed to anticipate convenience stores and 1,500-calorie fast-food meals. Fat is your energy supply, the fuel that feeds your internal furnace. If you don't use it, it will remain in storage. Only by using your muscles can you summon it from storage and burn it off. Thus you acquire and store fat unconsciously and with ease, but to get rid of it takes a conscious effort.

At the same time, you're up against thousands of years of technological advances. You may wish you were more active, but technology is pushing you in the other direction. Think of all the inventions in the last 50 years designed to make your life easier, shorten your workday, and lengthen your leisure hours or fill them with passive amusements. When's the last time you got up and walked the 10 feet between the couch and the television to change the channel instead of using the remote control? We have remote controls for everything from stereos and CD players to thermostats and air-conditioners. Push a button and the windows go down in the car. You don't even have to wind your watch any more. Need to carve the Thanksgiving turkey? Get out the electronic carving knife. Need to drive a screw? Use the battery-operated screwdriver. In a million little ways, every day, we save ourselves the trouble of exerting ourselves.

That's not necessarily a good thing.

All the labor-saving devices invented in the 1950s and 1960s, designed to "liberate" you from the drudgery of housework, have instead freed you to do housework *and* hold down a job outside the home. We are all busier than ever, multitasking from morning to midnight, the proverbial rat race carrying us along at a faster pace than ever before. The difference is that now all your exertion is mental. And too often, when you're done with a hard day's work, when you finally have a moment, you want something to soothe you, so you reach for what's closest at hand—most likely a high-calorie food or drink of dubious nutritional value.

What Is Appetite?

Is it in your mind, or in your stomach? Or does it come from someplace else entirely?

Appetite regulation is complicated, and involves both the brain and hormone signals from the gastrointestinal tract. The "appetite center" is located in the hypothalamus, part of the brain directly behind the eyes and on top of the pituitary gland, a very important part of the endocrine system. The hypothalamus is responsible for regulating a variety of systems in addition to appetite. It regulates your temperature and it coordinates the actions of the hormones involved in puberty.

In normal people, low blood sugar stimulates the appetite center in the hypothalamus to release "signals" that result in the sensation of hunger. After eating, other hormones released by the gastrointestinal tract send a signal that the brain senses as satiety, or fullness, telling the body it's time to stop eating. In some situations you do not "feel full" after eating. Some of these conditions can have a physical cause. Some children who undergo certain types of brain surgery or children born with Prader-Willi syndrome, a rare genetic disorder that results in profound obesity, lack what medical science believes to be normal appetite centers, and thus will not stop eating on their own.

Often people who overeat and disregard their satiety signals do so under emotional stress. Other individuals who have very high insulin levels (and who are insulin resistant) may experience frequent low blood sugar during the day that may alter the sensation of satiety. (For more on insulin resistance, see page 31)

Researchers have been trying for years to come up with a pill to cure obesity or control appetite. The most promising may be the work reported in the *New England Journal of Medicine*, of British scientists who injected volunteers at London's Hammersmith Hospital with a naturally occurring hormone called PYY, first discovered in pig intestines in 1980. Studies showed that subjects ate 30 percent less after being injected with PYY, which brings on a feeling of satiety. It's believed that obese people secrete less PYY than lean people. It will, however, be years before PYY can be brought to the marketplace as a potential treatment for obesity.

Your Children Are at Risk

It would be bad enough if it were just a problem for grown-ups, but the sad truth is that your children are subject to the same pressures and forces that affect you—and are probably even more vulnerable. At best, they eat the same foods you do, but most likely they eat worse than you do when they're on their own. And the same things that make you inactive make your kids inactive. They ride or take the bus to school, maybe because it's too far or too dangerous to walk or ride their bicycles. Across the country, schools facing budget constraints and under pressure to concentrate on math, English, and science, cut back on gym classes. In fact, according to a report by the National Association for Sport and Physical Education, only Illinois still requires daily physical education for all children up to 12th grade.

In many school districts, after-school programs have been cut, so kids may return to empty homes where they can snack and watch television or play video games.

Some schools have even contracted with soft drink companies or fast-food chains to furnish or supplement school lunches. School vending machines sometimes account for nearly a third of all on-campus food sales, claim Coca-Cola executives in a *New York Times* interview. And although many suppliers are offering to stock healthier foods alongside the cookies and potato chips, you don't have to be Nostradamus to predict which foods your children are likely to choose.

But in the pages ahead, you and your family will learn how to resist these forces and to choose healthy foods—and how to introduce daily activity and exercise into your lives.

How Long Will This Program Take?

Everyone wants to know.

Each of the seven workshops should be reinforced through practical applications. Your goal is to encourage adopting good habits without regard to schedules or deadlines. You live in an age (and a society) of instant gratification. Every day you probably see ads offering you pills or programs guaranteed to take off large amounts of weight quickly. Bookstores offer books outlining 10-minute fitness programs. Late-night cable infomercials depict electronic weight-loss devices that will supposedly lose weight *for you*—all you have to do is belt them on, press a button, close your eyes, and take a nap.

What you should take is a deep breath.

There's a great deal of wisdom to the old saying that if something sounds too good to be true, it probably is. Such quickie weight-loss schemes, ranging from marginally beneficial dietary supplements to old-fashioned quackeries and placebos to medically dangerous substances such as ephedra or Phen-fen all have one thing in common. They have selling power. Selling power is good for the manufacturers and the mail-order vendors.

What you really want is something that works, is safe, and has *staying* power.

So you shouldn't feel that you're in a race or a hurry to lose weight. It's normal to want to have a sense of progress, and to anxiously await results, but remember that everyone is going to progress at a different rate. Growing children are making progress if they simply stop *gaining* weight—because as they're growing taller, they're growing leaner. Turn off the clocks and throw away the calendars. Healthful habits should apply every day of the week, every week of the year. Set goals, but remember that while you will feel triumph and glory at reaching your goals, there is no moment when the achievement of your goals lets you resume your unhealthful activities.

"My daughter gained confidence and nutritional awareness."

—KidShape parent

You will be participating in one preliminary meeting (where you devise a reward system and take a basic fitness test) plus seven workshops. It will be up to you and your family to decide how much time to spend on each workshop. Some steps may take longer than others, and timing will vary from family to family. You could complete one workshop per week, or split each workshop up into two or more weeks. Many families find that the best approach is to commit two hours (or about the time it takes to watch a video) one day a week, perhaps on a Saturday afternoon, get as much as possible done during that session, and then schedule three exercise sessions for the rest of the week. The organizer will want to save time by preparing materials and photo-copies ahead of time.

Keep in mind that this is not a competition to see who in your family can lose the most weight, even though kids are often competitive and engage in sibling rivalries. Usually kids compete for one thing—your attention—so make sure each child knows he or she is going to be heard. While everyone may share the same overall goal, each person's specific aim is different. Parents or siblings who are not overweight may have goals such as increasing strength, increasing energy, or developing a healthier lifestyle. Your family is made up of unique individuals, with age, gender, and other differences. These differences will, to varying degrees, influence weight, strength, and body composition in childhood and throughout your lives.

Who Can Participate?

Parents often raise the question, who *can* participate? What they are really ask-ing is, who *should* participate? The simple answer is that the workshops are useful for anyone and everyone. It is not harmful to anyone to learn how to eat healthier, get more exercise, and feel better about oneself. So let's get to the real question: how do you know if your child needs to participate in a weight man-agement program? Even before starting the program, you should know your child's height and weight (if necessary, you can easily get this information from your child's doctor), and you can use this information to calculate your child's body mass index (see pages 44–46). If your child's BMI is above the 85th per-centile for age, your child really is overweight and would benefit from changes in diet and exercise habits.

Sometimes parents are not sure whether a child is emotionally affected by a weight problem. The child may seem unconcerned, so parents fear that by bringing up the issue, they will create a problem where there is none. To assess the situation, you can ask your child about teasing at school and about feelings about his or her body without particularly focusing on weight. Whether or not your child is concerned about weight, the issue needs to be dealt with for health reasons. The workshops will enable you to make simple changes for the whole family without pointing your finger at the overweight child.

At what age can children begin the program? Children get the most out of the workshops when they are old enough to write in their own journals, usually at age six or older. However, siblings as young as three or four can participate in many of the activities, as well as in the physical exercise sections. The program works best when all family members learn and exercise together, so all children who are old enough should participate. If siblings who do not have weight problems are resistant, they may be motivated by the reward system described on pages 43–44. Only by "signing on" can they earn prizes and rewards.

Unfortunately, sometimes parents disagree about the existence or severity of a weight problem in the family. If your spouse or partner denies there is a problem or doesn't want to participate in the workshops, you can begin on your own to help your family eat healthier and exercise more. When your partner sees that you and your children are feeling happier and more energetic, he or she may feel motivated to join in.

It's best to check with your health care provider before beginning any diet or exercise program, especially for children who are significantly obese or for adults over forty who may have other health problems.

WHAT PARENTS SHOULD KNOW

- *Only one-third of all kids living a mile or less from school walk to classes, according to a study reported in* Women and Health.

- *Today only about half of all middle schools and a quarter of all high schools require three full years of physical education, according to the* President's Council on Physical Fitness and Sports Research Digest. *Only 16 percent of girls still have daily physical education beyond the 11th grade, reports* Women and Health.

- *The average nine-year-old child watches 25 hours of television per week, according to a study published in the* Archives of Pediatrics and Adolescent Medicine.

⊘ *If a child is obese at age seven, that child has a 40 percent chance of remaining obese as an adult, warns a report in* Pediatric Clinics of North America. *For an obese adolescent, the risk of adult obesity rises to 70 percent.*

⊘ *Kids show a significant decline in daily activity levels as they mature, according to a U.S. Department of Health and Human Services National Children and Youth Fitness Study, with 18-year-olds expending only half the calories (proportional to body size) they expended at age six.*

⊘ *Eighty-five percent of all five-year-old children in the United States cannot pass a basic physical fitness test, finds a University of Minnesota at Minneapolis study.*

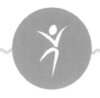

CHAPTER 2

The Family Table

The rise of obesity in the United States over the past 15 years is the result of several factors, all converging to form a "perfect storm" of cheap fatty foods, less physically demanding exercise, and more sedentary leisure and work-time activities.

But you don't have to change the whole environment for yourself or your family to start losing weight. All you have to do is change the environment *in your own home.* When you think of the benefits compared to the potential costs in terms of health, changing your home environment is clearly worth it.

At one time being overweight was considered a sign of affluence and not a health risk. Kids could see successful athletes such as Yankee great Babe Ruth or Chicago Bears defensive tackle William "The Refrigerator" Perry and think that you could be overweight and still be fit. Both men were successful athletes, but neither was fit. Ruth died at 53, and half of retired football players older than 50 have high blood pressure and heart disease—and those overweight linemen are three times more likely to have these conditions.

The fact is that being overweight is not benign. The medical evidence is overwhelming. A whopping *61 percent* of American adults are at risk for serious weight-related health problems, according to an article in the *International Journal of Obesity and Related Metabolic Disorders.* And these health problems kill 300,000 of us every year—second only to smoking, as reported in the *Journal of the American Medical Association.* Worldwide, the World Health Organization now blames obesity-related diseases for 30 million deaths annually.

Excessive weight contributes to or causes all these conditions:

→ Type 2 diabetes

→ Heart disease

→ Stroke

→ Hypertension

→ Gallbladder disease

→ Osteoarthritis

→ Fractures and bone malformation

→ Many types of cancer

→ High blood cholesterol

→ Heart and circulatory problems

→ Complications of pregnancy

→ Menstrual irregularities

→ Stress incontinence

→ Increased surgical risk and complications

→ Breathing problems such as asthma and sleep apnea

→ Fatty liver disease

Many of these disorders and illnesses—hypertension, type 2 diabetes, even heart disease—are more and more often turning up in children as young as three. Tragically, the longer a person has these diseases, the more damage they do, giving overweight kids a very dangerous "head start."

What Is Diabetes?

Diabetes mellitus is among the oldest diseases in recorded history. In Latin, the name literally means "honey-sweet urine," which refers to the passage of sugar in your urine. In diabetes, you suffer from inadequate insulin, the hormone that regulates your blood sugar levels.

Insulin is found even in the most primitive forms of life, from primitive sponges to the lowly hagfish and on up the food chain. Insulin is a protein, made by the pancreas, an organ that surrounds the stomach. Your pancreas releases insulin in response to eating and it influences your blood sugar after you eat by promoting the uptake of glucose by your muscle tissues. Insulin tells your body to take up the sugars from the blood and store fats for later use. Without insulin, the body breaks down stored fats, creating an excess of acidic compounds called ketones in the blood, which in turn increases respiration as the body strives to reduce the blood's acid content. A lack of insulin also allows sugar to build up in the blood, resulting in frequent urination and thirst. This excess blood sugar is what causes serious health problems.

In type 1 diabetes, which usually begins before age 19, you produce no insulin, and must take insulin by injection and carefully monitor your blood sugar levels and what you eat. In this type of diabetes the body's immune system attacks and destroys the cells in your pancreas that make insulin, and unfortunately it is not preventable or curable.

In type 2 diabetes the body either fails to produce enough insulin or cannot adequately use the insulin it has, because being overweight interferes with insulin action (this is known as insulin resistance). This type of diabetes has routinely been most common in overweight people over age 60, but now increasingly occurs in young people as well. About 80 percent of people with type 2 diabetes are overweight, and often losing weight and beginning to exercise can reverse this type of diabetes. Doctors may also prescribe pills that increase the secretion of insulin from the patient's pancreas or ones that increase sensitivity to their usual levels of insulin.

Physicians today have found an alarming increase in children as young as seven developing type 2 diabetes, a disease once limited to their grandparents. Diabetes is now the most expensive chronic disease in the United States. It is a truly disabling disease, partly because some people don't take it as seriously as it should be taken. (And many people have type 2 diabetes without being aware of it, so it's important to ask to be tested.) In both types of diabetes, it's important to keep blood sugar levels in the normal range. Without this, sugar can damage blood vessels and nerves, and can result in blindness, kidney failure, nerve damage, impotence, and poor blood flow to the extremities (fingers, toes, and feet) which may eventually require amputations. Ultimately, without good control of blood sugar and blood cholesterol, premature death can result from early occurrence of heart attacks and strokes.

Genetic factors can make you more prone to develop type 2 diabetes—but it certainly is not inevitable. The best treatment is a good offense: starting now to keep your weight at a healthy level, to eat well, and to stay active.

There's an emotional component and an emotional price as well, especially for overweight children, who are vastly more prone to suffer emotional difficulties and psychological syndromes. The truth is that children and sometimes adults torment fat children. And children with weight problems often grow up to be adults with serious health problems, who are in turn more likely to have overweight kids.

The Solution Is at Hand

You are the solution.

We know that early intervention is the surest way to alter unhealthy behaviors before they become entrenched habits. We know that kids need to be taught what those unhealthy behaviors are and how and why to change them, but too often, the teacher is a doctor or a dietitian or a school health-care worker. Too often, parents say, "Let's leave it to the experts."

But *you* are the expert. No one is in a better position to help children learn than their parents or family members. Parents influence their children's eating habits more than any other figure, according to a survey published in the *Journal of the American Dietetic Association.* You have powers you may not even be aware of. Family therapy has been applied successfully over the last 30 years to address a variety of problems, including eating disorders, substance abuse, delinquency, promiscuity, and other self-destructive behaviors. Often, kids choose these behaviors to express their feelings because they know no other way.

You can teach them another way. You start by sitting around the family table, eating together, listening to each other, and learning how you can change your environment and your lifestyle. This program works because it's not a diet, but a program for lifestyle change. In your family, the whole is stronger than the sum of its parts. The love you feel toward your children, and the love they feel for you and each other, are all resources you can call upon when the going gets tough. No other diet program has this!

Family therapy works well for overeating and obesity because kids frequently use food to express their feelings, particularly when overeating becomes a control issue. You may remember how hard it can be to get two-year-olds to eat, when the little darlings realize they can turn their heads or spit food out when the mood strikes them. Food is one of the few areas where kids have some control. Kids quickly realize they can get special considerations when they're sick and can become problem eaters as a way of obtaining the love they need: Food feels good immediately, and temporarily fills an empty place inside. Overeating becomes a symptom of something deeper within the family that needs to be addressed. Your parenting style may need to change first, to help your children learn to express themselves and know they're being listened to.

"It is important and necessary to take action when our children's health is at risk."

—KidShape parent

Your family doesn't have to resemble the *Father Knows Best* sitcom model for this approach to weight control to work for you. The makeup of families today is very different from families 50 years ago; many families include stepchildren or grandparents or involve shared custody. Whether you're a single parent with an only child or a two-parent household with a brood of 12, if you have a place to live and a table where you eat, you have what you need to get started.

Imagine, for a moment, the reverse. Think how difficult it would be for your child to try to work on his or her weight problem alone. A "fat camp" or after-school nutritional educational program may help temporarily, but at home the child is surrounded by all the reasons and means that led to overeating in the first place.

Why the Family Table Approach Works

Perhaps you're saying to yourself, "How can I help my *child* lose weight, when I can't even shed the 10 extra pounds *I'm* carrying around?"

If that describes you, remember that the support in the family approach is not a one-way street. Your child will be helping you almost as much as you'll be helping your child. A family approach wouldn't work if the child were the only one to get something out of it. There has to be something in it for everybody. In most cases, parents who help their children lose weight, also lose weight. Parental fitness levels improve, and the associated health issues improve too.

Why?

Because the family table approach you'll be taking relies on the relationships within your family to address individual problems. A family is webbed together in countless ways. Help one individual and the whole network benefits. Studies show that interactions among family members can affect health and well-being more quickly and permanently than interacting just with doctors or nutritionists. No doctor's authority can compete with the authority you have over your children, and no nutritionist's professional concern or approval can compete with the love you can give your child as motivation or reinforcement. When they return that love to you, you will find yourself motivated and your efforts reinforced in ways you hadn't thought possible, and you will find it easy to commit to the process—even if you found it difficult to commit to shedding your own excess weight before.

You can do more as a member of a team than you could ever do alone. That's true for you, and it's true for your kids. An individual generally becomes overweight as a result of family-wide poor eating and exercise habits. And that person often overeats in direct response to family pressures, which need to be addressed.

Treating a child without involving the whole family doesn't work. How much luck have you had, having one kid skip dessert when everyone else digs in? Singling out the overweight child only makes it worse. A healthy meal, with correct portion sizes, treats everyone fairly. When everyone in the family joins the same program, your overweight child will feel supported and free to share personal experiences at the table. The family table approach is not only the most effective approach but also the most supportive.

Weight loss is only one of the many benefits you'll see. Joining forces at the family table can help improve your family's communication skills and sometimes discipline methods. Your children, by learning to control their impulses and resist peer pressure, are learning skills that can help them avoid substance abuse when they become older. Eating and working together may even enhance your child's intellectual abilities. A study reported in the *Canadian Journal of Public Health* found that eating dinner together as a family increases a child's scores on the pre-SATs and the SATs. Other studies, such as one done by the California Department of Education, suggest that children involved in regular exercise earn better grades and have better social skills than those who don't exercise.

Physically, the benefits of losing weight are numerous. Eating right and exercising helps build and maintain muscles, joints, and bones and reduces the risk of cancer, hypertension, diabetes, heart disease, and premature death. Emotionally, the results are obvious. Your children will be stronger, more attractive, feel more liked by their peers, and feel better about themselves. It won't hurt either when the compliments start coming in, when friends and others notice that they've lost weight.

Taking One Step at a Time

You've already taken the first step. Recognizing the problem is often difficult. Even for those of us who suspect a problem, it's altogether too easy to do nothing, to deny the problem, justify it, rationalize it, or hope it will go away on its own.

Committing to making a change is the second step—and it's considerably easier when love is the motivating force. Actively seeking health and fitness for you and your family is a profoundly loving thing to do. It's difficult for any of us to make lifestyle and behavioral changes alone, particularly children. It takes a whole family to counter that isolation and reduce the effects of stigmatization.

The third step is realizing that while change can be frightening, the anticipation of change is what's intimidating, not the change itself. Returning to the family table won't be arduous or unpleasant. If your family already maintains a routine of eating together, bringing the subject of weight loss and exercise to the table will only require tweaking something you already enjoy. Getting in shape doesn't have to be a rigorous program—it can be as simple as borrowing the neighbor's dog to walk—and it can be lots of fun. The key is developing a network of family and friends and becoming physically active together.

Remember that the causes of overweight and obesity are varied, and in many ways indeed a response to our environment. Blame could be distributed among the schools, food companies, economy, technology, passive entertainment, indolent culture, unsafe playgrounds, and rise of spectator sports over participatory activities, all factors that have been ganging up against us for the last 30 years. But a family, working together, can cut through all these factors to a new, healthy way of life.

The bottom line is this: Anyone who has ever tried to lose weight knows that one of the hardest parts is the loneliness, the sense that you're on your own, fighting your impulses. Hunger is, by definition, an internal feeling, a private craving that starts deep in your gut. Hunger turns our focus inward, seizes our attention, and makes us lonely. We eat, in part, to not feel that way. By addressing a weight problem at the family table, your overweight child will feel less alone. Your mere presence at the table will reduce your son or daughter's loneliness, and in turn reduce the number of calories desired. You may find you feel less alone too, or less helpless.

Here are two stories that may give you an idea of what you can expect to achieve in your own home. Note that while you won't be meeting with nutritionists, mental health professionals, or physical trainers, the tools provided in this book will enable you to write your own success story.

KEVIN'S STORY

Roberta and her husband, Larry, became concerned when they noticed a bump on the neck of their eight-year-old, Kevin, near the top of his spine. At first Roberta thought it was because he had poor posture from spending too much time hunched over, playing with his Game Boy. He'd never been an active child, primarily because he was afraid of a mean dog next door, so he watched cartoons instead.

Kevin's pediatrician could not identify the problem but referred him to a pediatric endocrinologist, who diagnosed the child immediately.

"Your child is overweight," she said. "The bump on Kevin's neck is called a 'buffalo hump.' They're fairly common among people struggling with a weight problem."

Roberta had never regarded her son as overweight, although she realized that he had always been self-conscious. "I noticed he was always tugging at his shirt to cover his belly," she said. "And he'd cried once and said he didn't want to go to school because kids teased him, but he wouldn't tell me why they teased him. I didn't want to press him on it so I just let it go."

Even though Kevin ate relatively healthy meals with his family, he snacked on chips while doing his homework, and drank the soda that was always in the refrigerator. Roberta realized that she'd always used food as a reward or incentive to do something. One of Kevin's favorite places to go was Chuck E. Cheese, for pizza slathered in melted cheese. Other times they'd go to all-you-can-eat buffets.

Kevin and his parents attended a two-hour session every weekend. They met with a nutritionist for 30 minutes, and then a mental health professional for 30 minutes, where they talked about the emotional issues underlying Kevin's eating. For the last hour, Kevin worked with the trainer and other kids, playing games and doing exercises designed to be fun. The nutritionist recommended sliced apples or carrots for Kevin to snack on instead of chips, explaining that he was craving something crunchy.

Kevin and his mom and dad learned how to read nutrition labels on foods. "I'd watch him out of the corner of my eye and see him pick things up and read the backs of the labels and then put the high-calorie items back on the shelves," Roberta says. "I didn't even have to say anything to him. He decided what he wanted on his own." When Kevin realized how many calories were in a Big Mac, he was excited to realize that by skipping the Big Mac, he could have a lot of other foods instead.

Roberta thinks the program works because it involves kids instead of telling them what to do. "It lets them take charge of their own weight and health, by teaching them how to be conscious of what they are eating."

Now when the ice cream truck comes to Kevin's school, he gets the fruit-flavored sorbet instead of ice cream. Roberta is more conscious of what foods she buys, serving chicken for dinner, with red meat no more than twice a week. She stocks fruits and veggies instead of chips, soda, and juice, and cooks vegetables that her son likes, such as broccoli, cauliflower, and sometimes cabbage. Now, as a reward or incentive, Kevin chooses between going to Chuck E. Cheese or spending the same amount of money at Toys R Us. So far, he has decided to go with the toys, specifically a basketball, football, and skateboard.

The entire family has become much healthier. Even Larry, who had been health conscious and worked out regularly, lost 10 pounds. Kevin lost 6 pounds while growing two inches taller—the equivalent of losing 14 pounds. Now when Roberta looks at Kevin, she sees a much happier boy, one who really likes being in control of what he is eating.

"He came home one day," Roberta reports, "and he had a big smile on his face because that day two people had told him he was looking better. 'Can you really tell, Mama?' he asked me. He needed to hear it from other people because he had a hard time seeing the difference when he just looked in the mirror."

GABRIELLA'S STORY

Marcia's five-year-old daughter, Gabriella, was in the habit of finishing her dinner and asking for a sandwich before going to bed. Marcia gave in although she knew Gabriella shouldn't be hungry, but didn't want to make Gabriella go to bed hungry. Gabriella knew she was overweight and wanted to do something about it because kids at school were picking on her and calling her fat. Being called names made her feel really bad.

Marcia started working with Gabriella when she turned six, although Marcia was concerned that some of the information being provided by the doctors and nutritionists was going to be over her head. Within the first three weeks, Gabriella began to catch on. After learning how to read the fat grams and total calories per servings on food labels, Gabriella began to lose weight. She drank water instead of juice and soda. She learned how the body turns crackers into starch, which is then turned into sugars. She learned that she does not have to clean her plate if she is not hungry. The best part of the program was when she got to play outside, with other kids who didn't tease her. She did push-ups and jumping jacks and felt herself getting stronger and stronger.

"The thing I liked about the program was that the doctors explained that it was not a diet, but more a chance to teach kids at an early age how to eat healthfully," Marcia says. "I was amazed at how quickly Gabriella picked up the information."

She admits that she picked up some useful information herself, discovering ways she could change her own lifestyle to make her family healthier.

"I was working long hours as a neurosurgeon's administrative assistant, and sometimes I'd get home so late that all I could do was grab a bag of food at McDonald's on my way home. I'd gained 20 pounds myself because I never took time to cook except on weekends. Now, I'll make up a menu for the whole week on Saturday and decide what we're going to have every day. Then I'll shop for the whole week, prepare meals beforehand, and put labeled packages in the freezer."

Now Gabriella tells Marcia what she can or can't eat, and her favorite food has become apples, with carrots a close second. Now when Marcia suggests McDonald's, Gabriella chooses Subway or The Baja Grill, a Mexican restaurant that uses fresh ingredients and grills everything. Recently, Gabriella told her mom that she thinks she wants to make every day a healthy day.

Marcia and Gabriella exercise together. They started by walking uphill to a park about a mile from their house, a steep climb in the canyons.

"Gabriella used to cry and beg me to stop halfway up," Marcia reports. "Now she's hardly winded, and she loves walking the trails and identifying the plants she sees. And I'd have to say that I think the best part is that kids aren't picking on her at school anymore. People began to notice Gabriella's weight loss almost immediately and saying nice things. And she has a new friend she might not have had the courage to meet before. She likes school now, where before, she dreaded it. Before, she wouldn't let people see her cry when they teased her about her weight, and would save her tears for when she got home. She's happy now."

By the time Gabriella finished the eight-week program, she'd lost 12 pounds, dropping from 73 pounds to 61 pounds which, because she was closer to a seven- or eight-year-old in height, was her appropriate weight.

WHAT PARENTS SHOULD KNOW

- The number of overweight children and adolescents in America has tripled over the last 40 years, and 15 million children over the age of five are now overweight, as reported in the Archives of Pediatric and Adolescent Medicine.

- Ten million young people in America today, one out of every six, are at risk for serious, life-limiting, and even life-threatening health problems, warns The Surgeon General's Call to Action to Prevent and Decrease Overweight and Obesity.

- A University of Minnesota at Minneapolis study found that 26 percent of overweight kids who were teased at school about their weight considered suicide, and 36 percent of the girls and 19 percent of the boys reported being depressed.

- You are the strongest role model for your children: Twenty-three percent of children ages 8 to 12 state that their mothers are their primary role models and 17.4 percent name their fathers as their primary role models, reports a study in the journal Childhood Education. Only 8.3 percent named celebrities.

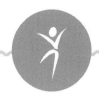

CHAPTER 3

The Truth behind Food Myths

Before starting the workshops, let's first dispel a few common beliefs about diet and exercise. It's important to separate myth from fact when it comes to food and nutrition. Some of the myths we grow up with lead us to being overweight or unhealthy.

MYTH #1:
Children Grow Out of Being Fat

The Myth: A chubby baby is a healthy baby. Being over-weight as a child isn't really a problem, because eventually children grow out of their baby fat. Worrying about a child's weight is just a form of vanity.

The Facts: While it's true that being overweight affects appearance, the related health problems go much deeper. You're not being vain if you worry about your child's weight. You're being a good parent. Children who are overweight can grow into adults with serious, even life-threatening health problems. It's true that doctors and parents look for and welcome a robust appetite in a newborn, when latching on and learning to breast-feed is important. A lack of weight gain in the first few weeks or months can be cause for concern, and of course, parents worry whether their child is getting enough nutrition as new foods are introduced and accepted or rejected. Everybody wants to see a baby with a healthy appetite.

It can be difficult to know when you should be concerned about your child's size. Asking your pediatrician is always a good idea. The accepted medical definition of "overweight" is when a child's body mass index (BMI) is above the 85th percentile for children the same age and sex (see pages 226 and 228). "Obesity" is defined when the BMI exceeds the 95th percentile for age and sex. When growth is normal, children exhibit rates of height and weight gain that follow the normal growth curves (see pages 227 and 229). Your child's physician keeps copies of these charts as a way of tracking changes. Generally doctors become concerned if a child gains more than 10 pounds in a year after the third birthday.

Practically speaking, however, no time is too early for you to be aware of your child's weight. (Note, however, that you should not serve low-fat milk to a child under the age of two, because fat is an important nutrient for developing children.)

MYTH #2:
Being Overweight is Biological Destiny

The Myth: Being overweight is caused by hormones, genetics, and other things that can't be changed.

The Facts: Medical science has identified several physiological causes of being overweight, but that doesn't mean there's nothing you and your family can do to counteract them.

Hormones do regulate a wide range of body processes, including growth and how your body uses and stores nutrients, and they affect your weight and energy level. The most powerful weight-regulating hormone is insulin, a chemical the body releases into the blood when you eat. Insulin regulates how fast you use fats, starches, and carbohydrates, and tells your body to use the food you've just eaten instead of your fat stores. Insulin also helps your cells store extra nutrients for later use.

In diabetes, a lack of insulin lets sugars build up in the blood. Insulin resistance, which can lead to type 2 diabetes, may occur in some people who chronically eat too much or snack constantly, causing their bodies to produce more insulin than their cells can handle. The cells become more resistant to insulin to fend off the surplus, and in return, the body senses that resistance and produces more insulin to compensate. Insulin resistance results from a genetic predisposition, poor diet, and a lack of exercise—the latter two factors can be modified by changes in lifestyle.

Hormonal conditions are not destiny.

Neither are genes. You probably know families where every member is tall and lean, or where every member is short and stocky. Like hormones, genes affect height, weight, and body shape. But you can be fit, no matter what body type you were born with. While genes can contribute to your build and weight, environment is the stronger influence. You teach your children how to eat, how to choose food, how to prepare it, how to serve it, when to serve it, how fast to eat it, how to savor it, how to feel about it, what to do after they eat, and what to do between meals. Family has everything to do with how and what we eat and how much exercise we get.

Where your body is concerned, you are the captain of your own ship. Even if your family does have some physiological or genetic component that contributes to being overweight, that's all the more reason to eat and exercise in a healthy way now.

MYTH #3:
Some People Are Overweight for No Reason

The Myth: Some people are just big-boned, or have slow metabolisms.

The Facts: Just as you can probably think of families where everyone is tall and lean, or short and stocky, you can probably also think of someone you know who apparently can eat anything she wants without gaining a pound. Or someone who seems to gain two pounds every time he eats an ice cream cone. The odds are probably good that the former is more active than she realizes, and the latter more sedentary than he wants to admit. Even so, people are different, with an endless variety of body types.

In the same way, we all have different metabolisms. "Metabolic rate" is how fast your body uses your food for fuel. People with slower metabolic rates burn less of the calories they eat and store the rest as fat; people with faster metabolisms burn more of the calories they take in and store very little as fat. While people with fast metabolisms tend to be naturally leaner, those with slow metabolisms are by no means condemned to being overweight. Your metabolic rate is influenced by several factors including age, sex, the presence of fever, the environmental temperature, your muscle mass, your hormone levels (particularly insulin and hormones produced by the thyroid), and your sensitivity to these hormones. The most important influence is exercise, which kicks your metabolism into high gear by telling it to burn that extra fuel that your body has stored as fat. In addition, you can increase your muscle mass by strength training, which further increases your metabolic rate.

Any body shape or metabolism has an appropriate weight range. No one is overweight for "no reason." Most people have more than one reason why they're overweight. The key to losing weight is understanding those reasons—which this book will explain.

MYTH #4:
By Instinct, Children Know When to Stop Eating

The Myth: Children know instinctively when they've had enough to eat.

The Facts: Most children up to age three know when to stop eating, but beyond this age children are as likely to overeat as adults, and in most cases are more susceptible to the pressures adults feel.

You already know the primal instinct a parent feels about feeding a child. You wanted to protect and nurture your newborn. As your child got older, the baby books told you to introduce one new food at a time and be on the lookout for allergic reactions. "They'll tell you what they want to eat and what they don't," your own parents may have advised. When you were in doubt, you perhaps overfed your baby, reasoning that it was better than underfeeding. "Eating is a natural process," you may have told yourself. "The baby will tell me what to do."

It doesn't really work that way—children tend to lack impulse control, and when you factor in the cute toys packaged with child meals at fast-food restaurants, the notion that children should somehow "naturally" resist eating too much high-calorie or tasty food seems a little wishful.

It's more logical to assume that our instincts would tell us to gorge ourselves when food is plentiful, feasting in anticipation of future famine. We developed as social animals, and among social animals the most aggressive at

What Birth Weight Can Mean

Sometimes parents are proud when their newborn debuts at a whopping 10 pounds, and worried when one weighs much less. While both can be perfectly healthy children, it's good to realize that babies who are more than nine pounds at birth or less than six pounds have a higher risk of being obese in the future.

Here's why. Big babies have formed metabolic paths that promote storing nutrients as fat, instead of burning them for energy. Small babies are playing "catch up" to reach normal size and weight, and most of them do this by their second birthday. Their bodies have been storing calories for growth, instead of burning them for energy, and if this mechanism persists, these stored "growth" calories become stored fat.

Forewarned can be forearmed, so if your child was born at a high or low weight, you may want to be especially careful with family meal planning and to be sure to incorporate regular exercise into family life.

getting the most food stands the best chance of surviving. Think of wolves or lions fighting with each other over food, driven by their instincts for self-preservation. Humans are, of course, considerably more polite, but we have some of the same instincts.

Your children don't instinctively know when to stop eating, certainly not past the toddler phase. In a Penn State study, three-year-olds stopped eating when they were full regardless of how much was served. Five-year-olds, however, polished off super-sized platefuls of macaroni and cheese (far more than a serving size) almost every time.

Children, however, can be taught when to stop eating and how to know when to stop. They can learn what it feels like to be full and what constitutes a serving, as well as how to identify emotional eating, mindless snacking, and compulsive eating.

MYTH #5:
Dieting Makes Children Unhappy

The Myth: Putting kids on diets only makes them feel bad about themselves and increases the risk of eating disorders.

The Facts: Kids who are obese or overweight are already unhappy, rating their own happiness at approximately the same level as kids with cancer undergoing chemotherapy, according to a University of California at San Diego study. In fact, most overweight people are to varying degrees unhappy. Kids often learn to mask their unhappiness by joking about their weight, struggling to compensate for a constant inner sadness. Some overeat because they're unhappy, while others are unhappy because they're too heavy. But lifestyle changes that lead to healthier eating and more exercise will positively affect both physical and emotional states.

Exercise helps improve mood and mental health in a variety of ways. Depression is usually reduced beginning as early as the very first exercise session, and depression continues to lessen as the child works out harder and longer. Many studies have shown that exercise is effective at treating anxiety and depression.

Exercise also produces better sleep patterns. People who exercise sleep longer hours and experience deeper, more recuperative, and more restorative kinds of sleep. And, of course, exercise improves muscle tone, strengthens heart and lungs, and can help make your child more flexible.

The joy kids feel when they lose weight is sincere and real. You'll know by the smiles on their faces. But change invites resistance. Initiating a fitness program will probably create a certain amount of griping. All of that is natural, and quite temporary. Your kids will soon learn that they're not trapped in a rigorous regimen requiring enormous willpower or self-deprivation. Meeting together to learn and exercise will enable your family to work as its own support group.

MYTH #6:
Dieting Leads to Poor Nutrition

The Myth: Restricting what we eat will make us unhealthy and maybe even restrict the children's growth.

The Facts: Some diets *can* lead to a nutritional imbalance, if they completely eliminate or drastically reduce one or more food groups. These kinds of diets could indeed be harmful to growing children and are not recommended.

That's not what you'll be doing. When you meet at the family table, you will be educating your children about the importance of balanced menus and controlled portion sizes. The whole point is to assure good nutrition by showing your kids the difference between healthy foods and unhealthy foods, and teaching them how to substitute fresh fruits and vegetables for junk food, high-fiber grain foods for low-fiber ones, and low-fat proteins for the usual fatty fare. You'll be showing them how to take smaller portions of the foods that are tempting but unhealthy and larger portions of the foods they truly need. You'll also be showing them how to stay active in a way that's fun and rewarding.

This is the path to health, not to malnutrition.

MYTH #7:
Popular Culture Will Win Out

The Myth: It's a losing battle and a waste of time—our entire family is bombarded with ads and other messages promoting junk food, and we can't stop our kids from watching TV or being influenced by pop culture.

The Facts: It's only a losing battle if you choose not to join the winning side.

Yes, popular culture will always be there, tempting you with easy pleasures and instant gratification, bombarding you with ads. But there's a way to live smart in such a world, both for you and for your kids.

Culturally, the messages are indeed insidious. Food companies air commercials aimed at kids during the early-morning or late-afternoon cartoon shows. Cartoon characters now appear on food packages, with SpongeBob SquarePants or Blue's Clues macaroni and cheese products, and even Sesame Street characters on high-calorie juice boxes. Checkout aisles at supermarkets offer candy and sugar products where kids shopping with their mothers can whine for the things they've seen advertised (but you can often select special "candy-free" checkouts). In the cereal aisle, you can see that the sugary cereals designed to appeal to children are at a child's eye level, while the healthy plain cereals are on the top shelf.

> *"The focus is on nutrition, not weight loss, and my daughter really got into it. She was really able to understand the information and is motivated."*
>
> —KidShape parent

But even if your children see an hour's worth of commercials every day, you still have 23 hours a day to counteract that message. Contrary to popular belief, your kids still listen to you more than they listen to the television. And if you limit the amount of television they watch, you'll limit the commercials they see as well.

The best place to engage the enemy is at the family table, where you are in charge of calorie content and portion sizes. (Obviously, you also must control what groceries you select and bring home.) Culture isn't destiny. By teaching your kids to resist the pressures of fast food, junk food, advertising, television, and passive entertainment, you can support and not sabotage your children's efforts. In this book you will also learn ways to deal with your feelings of guilt about your kids' weight and eating problems and ways to make positive changes in your homes and your communities to support healthy choices.

Remember, you have more influence over your child than a commercial— and, ultimately, you control what they eat and what they want to eat.

WHAT PARENTS SHOULD KNOW

Your best resource for information is your family doctor or pediatrician. Unfortunately, some parents are reluctant to bring up the subject of weight gain with their pediatrician, perhaps feeling it isn't important enough to mention or that they will be blamed for a child's weight (or that the doctor would of course mention it if it were a problem). Doctors may not bring it up for fear of alienating the family, or because they don't have the resources needed to address such a time- and staff-intensive problem, or just because they don't have a good solution and feel helpless. But weight gain is a legitimate health concern that can lead to serious problems. Some doctors, when faced with obese patients, lack sympathy, lose patience, or let their frustration show, but you can overcome such unprofessional behavior.

First, become an educated and proactive medical consumer, for your children and for yourself. Be candid and direct with your doctor. Talking to your doctor and getting referrals to specialists, endocrinologists, or dietitians should be covered by your health care provider. Many questions have complicated answers, so you should feel free to ask. Your questions may include the following:

1. *How do you know what's considered overweight in a child or adolescent, and how does that differ from adult standards?*

2. *What kinds of tests (such as x-rays, blood tests) can doctors do for children, or for adults, to determine what medical conditions may be concurrent with a person's obesity (such as hypertension, diabetes, coronary heart disease, stroke,*

gallbladder disease, osteoarthritis, sleep apnea) and how should a parent ask for additional tests?

3. How can you tell the difference between normal growth spurts and unhealthy weight gain in a growing child?

4. How can parents fill out and keep growth charts for their children, or for themselves?

5. How aggressive should parents be in getting medically supervised help for their child to lose weight, when the medical problems associated with obesity may complicate the weight loss process? How can a child with asthma or diabetes be more active without making things worse?

6. How can you tell when being overweight is so serious that it needs medical intervention?

7. How can you tell if a child has emotional problems commonly associated with being overweight, including eating disorders, anxiety, and depression?

8. How can you find information on specialists who are qualified to treat these problems, and where can you get advice on when, where, and how to seek professional help?

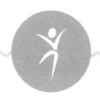

CHAPTER 4

Getting Started:
The First Meeting

At the First Meeting you will discuss what you're about to undertake as a family. This should not be a surprise meeting, but a time to come together to talk over how everybody feels about starting a weight loss program. Everyone should have adequate advanced notice. You may want to tell your kids something like, "Don't schedule anything next Monday evening, because we're going to have a family conference about starting a weight loss and fitness program together."

You will also talk about coming together to eat healthy, balanced, nutritious meals; exercising regularly; developing a "credit" system to develop incentives for each person's success. You will take a fitness test and do a little math to determine body mass index (BMI) for everyone, so you may want a simple calculator on hand.

You should decide when to have your regular meetings. For some families, it's simplest to meet at the same time every week. Meeting on weekday evenings can cut into homework time during the school year. Saturdays or Sundays after breakfast or lunch seems to work for most families.

Supplies and Materials You'll Need

Before the preliminary meeting, you will need to make copies of the materials in Appendix 1 (pages 216–241); look at the list on pages 213–215 to determine how many copies of each page you need. The quantities given for the weekly forms are guidelines only, based on completing the workshops in seven weeks. If your family takes longer, you will need additional copies of the weekly materials. You can photocopy the pages directly from the book or print out larger-size versions (8½ x 11 inches) from the KidShape Web site at www.kidshape.com. If you wish, you can photocopy or print the pages onto three-hole-punched paper (or use a three-hole punch to make the holes). You may also wish to use color paper for photocopying the food cards on pages 234–239 (for Workshop 3); note that if you have a color printer, you can print these in color from the Web site.

A fun way to begin the program might be a family field trip to the nearest office supply or discount store. Each participant will need something to write with and a folder or an inexpensive half-inch or one-inch three-ring binder (if you are using three-hole-punched paper) to hold the contract, questionnaires, logs, journal pages, and assorted materials you have photocopied.

At the store, your children should also pick out their favorite small stickers, to be used during the program to mark their achieved goals. Stickers appeal to most children, and the process of applying them to the chart is fun and provides a visual acknowledgment of a goal achieved. For those who prefer not to use stickers (such as adults), that's okay too.

On your shopping trip, you can also have each family member select a special water bottle to use when exercising.

Once you have all the supplies, hand the pages and stickers out and ask each person to store them in his or her folder or binder. Kids may enjoy decorating their own folders or binders. If only one copy of a form is needed for the entire family (such as the Family Reward Chart), a parent can store it.

While you're certainly welcome to use computers to keep journals and so on, we strongly recommend keeping paper printouts. Too often, computer files are lost or damaged. For kids, losing the records of all their hard work can be a crushing blow.

You'll also need an accurate bathroom scale (you can check yours with a five-pound sack of flour, a weight from a weight-lifting set, or a dumbbell) and a yardstick or tape measure to take an accurate reading of everyone's height. You'll need a watch with a second hand or a digital watch with a stopwatch function. Only multiplication and division is required, but a simple calculator will come in handy. Most computers also have calculator functions. Finally, though you won't need these items right away, you will need a food scale to weigh your food portions, measuring cups, measuring spoons, clear plastic sandwich bags, and a large can of shortening, such as Crisco.

To summarize, here are the supplies you will need for the workshops:

→ Photocopies or printouts of forms on pages 216–241 (see list on pages 213–215)

→ Three-hole punch or three-hole-punched paper (optional)

→ Colored paper for photocopying food cards (optional)

→ Folder or three-ring binder (half-inch or one-inch) for each participant

→ Small stickers

→ Water bottle for each participant (optional)

→ Scissors

→ Accurate bathroom scale

→ Yardstick or tape measure

→ Watch with a second hand or digital watch with stopwatch function

→ Calculator

→ Food scale

→ Measuring cups and measuring spoons

→ Clear plastic sandwich bags

→ Large can of shortening, such as Crisco

The Basics

Have an adult facilitate the First Meeting, but you're free to alternate or rotate the leadership at subsequent meetings. Before the First Meeting, the leader should become familiar with the charts referenced in this chapter, so he or she can explain them to other family members and answer their questions. Each workshop begins with a family meeting. The facilitator may also be called the coach, captain, or any other term your family chooses. Like a football coach in front of a team, the leader needs to explain what the family goals are and how they are to be met.

Everyone should first talk about why your family needs to change the way it eats and exercises. Describe the program in general terms and explain the format of each family workshop, which will begin with a discussion after reading the main topic. From the second workshop on, you'll briefly review the previous lesson. Then time will be set aside for talking and sharing feelings, problems, and triumphs. In each workshop, you'll set goals and monitor your progress. You'll all have homework assignments, designed to put into action what you're learning. At the end of each workshop, you will stretch for 10 minutes and then exercise for 30 more minutes, but if discussions take too long, you can schedule future exercise sessions. At the end of each period of physical activity, everyone should drink a glass of water—if you purchased new water bottles, this is the time to use them. All decisions should be made by the whole family and should receive full group support. You should explain why the family is doing this together—that it's easier for a team to accomplish a goal than it is for an individual, and far harder when only one member of a team is trying to effect change.

The Contract

Today you all need to read and sign the contract on page 224 (it is among the pages you photocopied and passed out, and should be in everyone's folder). Most children don't want to be left out. If a child says he or she doesn't want to participate, explain to them that no one can receive rewards unless they sign the contract. Parents may want to talk to an overweight child beforehand to make sure they don't feel singled out or stigmatized.

Devising a Reward System

Now comes the fun part—deciding how credit will be given and rewarded. The primary goal is to become healthier and feel better, but that's a little too vague and abstract for younger children to understand. You can measure weight loss on a bathroom scale and with a tape measure, and a doctor can measure improvements in blood pressure and cholesterol levels in a doctor's office, but children need something easier to envision as a positive reinforcement.

Food should *never* be used a reward. The cost of the rewards will vary, depending on your family budget, but some of them should be things that promote a more healthy lifestyle. A certain number of points might earn a Frisbee, a volleyball, a jump rope, a tennis racket, a CD to dance to, a scooter, or a bicycle. Activities may be used as rewards too, ranging from a walk to the park or a trip to the zoo or any other form of time with Mom and Dad. Money should never be used as a reward, because experience has shown that paying kids to lose weight doesn't work.

Bearing these things in mind, each participant should write down 10 things they want, ranging from small things to larger, more expensive ones. It may be easier if everybody writes down 20 things and then, perhaps with help from parents, whittles the list down to 10. When you've done that, rank them from 1 to 10 from smallest to largest.

Now look at the Weekly Point Chart on page 222 (it should be in each participant's folder) and review the list of things that points will be awarded for. At the beginning of each workshop, each participant will fill out this form. You may, if you wish, modify this list to suit your own family's needs—for example, you could include points for helping with housework, completing schoolwork, or practicing the piano, on the line for "additional points" on the chart.

Now see how to keep track of everyone's accumulated points, using the Family Reward Chart on page 223. You will also need to arrange each individual's list of rewards on a list and assign point values to them, where a walk in the park with Mom or Dad costs 50 points, a new CD costs 100, a skateboard costs 200, a new bicycle costs 300, and so on. Keep in mind that families may share points. For example, if a trip to Six Flags is worth 1,000 points, you could all pool points for this family trip. If you wish to allow kids to cash in points along the way (instead of at the end of the workshops), keep track of the deductions and what they were used for on the Family Reward Chart.

When certain behaviors are rewarded, they tend to continue. When good behaviors aren't recognized, your kids may stop them. While being healthy is in a sense its own reward, kids need more tangible reinforcements.

Taking a Baseline Measurement

The next thing is to reach an accurate diagnosis of the current starting point for everyone. All family members should fill out the Information Survey on page 225 (it should be in each participant's folder). Remember that there are no right or wrong answers, and you're not going to be graded or judged. You will not even be asked to share your questionnaires with others, though you are free to do so if you choose. The more honest you are with your answers, the more helpful this questionnaire is going to be. Family members may move to a more private location or separate room while they fill out this form. You may need to explain some of the questions to younger children, but children should complete the questionnaire on their own after it has been explained to them.

Fixing a starting point is complicated by the fact that childhood is, by definition, a time of growth. All children gain weight as their bones and muscles develop. When a child is overweight, balancing normal growth and weight gain with necessary weight loss can be tricky.

The best measure will be your child's BMI or body mass index, a figure used to help determine total body fat. Bear in mind that two people who are both five feet five and weigh 225 pounds will have the same BMI, even if one is obviously corpulent and the other is a bodybuilder with massive musculature. Your child's BMI is only one indicator. In order to determine everyone's BMI, you'll need to first measure height and weight. Be sure to take your shoes off first. You may want to weigh yourselves in your underwear for a more accurate reading.

When you've finished, you'll have to do a little bit of math. Divide your weight (in pounds) by your height (in inches) squared (multiplied by itself).

Then multiply the result by 703. If you have Internet access, you can use the automated BMI calculator at www.powerofprevention.com. Just enter the height, weight, age, and sex of each person, and the program will calculate the BMI and indicate whether it falls in the normal or abnormal range.

Why Some Overweight Children Are Tall

Some overweight children are taller than they should be. That is because, in some cases, children have converted the extra calories they consume into premature growth as well as girth, and become taller than normal. Parents are often pleased by this, but not when the child begins puberty early, another result of overeating. To find the predetermined genetic average height for boys, add together the parents' heights in inches, plus 5 inches, and divide by 2. For girls, add the parents' heights, minus 5 inches, and divide by 2.

Thus a boy whose mother is 5 feet 2 inches tall (62 inches) and whose father is 5 feet 6 inches tall (66 inches) would be expected to grow to 5 feet 6½ inches (62 + 66 + 5 = 133 inches; divided by 2 = 66½). You can then use the Stature-for-Age and Weight-for-Age Percentiles Charts for Boys (see page 227) to determine what the boy's height and weight should be at age 10. On the top right of the chart, where it says "stature," find the expected adult height of 66½ inches. Then follow the grid lines to the left to find the percentile: 66½ inches is between the 10th and 25th percentiles. If we follow along that growth curve, we see that when the boy is 10, he should be about 52 inches tall (4 feet 4 inches), if he is growing normally. The boy's weight (shown on the bottom of the chart) should also be between the 10th and 25th percentile, or an average of 60 pounds. However, if he is overweight, he may be 4 feet 8 inches tall and weigh 90 pounds, which is far above his expected height and weight.

This method makes it easy to see how much overeating has affected growth and how it may alter final height. If you have any doubts or questions about this assessment, contact your child's health care provider.

What Do the Numbers Mean?

When you're done, get the appropriate charts from your folder: Body Mass Index-for-Age Percentiles (Boys or Girls), Stature-for-Age and Weight-for-Age Percentiles (Boys or Girls), and Body Mass Index Table (Adults). (Charts are on pages 226–230.) In the box in the upper left corner of each chart, write down the date and your age, weight, stature (height), and BMI. You'll want those numbers for later comparison.

For men and women over age 20, if your BMI is less than 18.5, you're considered underweight. Between 18.5 and 24.9 is considered normal; 25 to 29.9 is overweight; 30 to 39.9 is obese, and 40 or higher is extremely obese.

Use the boys' and girls' charts to determine what percentile your child fits into according to BMI and stature. Normal is considered to fall between the 5th and 85th percentiles.

If these growth curves seem complicated, you may also consult your pediatrician. Most people can easily use them after some practice. If you have trouble, take two rulers or two straight-edged pieces of paper and line them up along the x and y axes to guide your eye. You can use these charts to determine your target weight by cross-referencing the BMI in the 18.5 to 24.9 range for your height and weight.

Calorie Intake and Ideal Body Weight

Your BMI will tell you approximately what your ideal weight is, but it doesn't tell you how many calories you need to eat each day to get there or to stay there. Ultimately all weight loss programs, whether trendy new diets or old standbys, are a matter of adjusting the ratio of calories taken in to calories burned.

You need to take in calories every day to maintain body functions, repair cells, provide materials for tissue growth and replacement, and to meet your energy demands. Your nutritional requirement is called your "basal energy expenditure," and it's based on your ideal body weight. On average, you need to eat about 15 calories for every pound you weigh to maintain your ideal weight, though if you're extremely active, training for a marathon, for instance, you'd need more, and if you're extremely inactive, you'd need less.

But what's your ideal weight?

IDEAL BODY WEIGHTS FOR ADULTS

Height (inches)	Healthy weight range (pounds)
58	88–119
59	91–123
60	95–127
61	98–132
62	101–136
63	104–140
64	108–145
65	111–149
66	114–154
67	118–159
68	121–163
69	125–168
70	129–173
71	132–178
72	136–183
73	140–188
74	144–194
75	148–199
76	152–204

Table 4.1

Souce: *Clinical Guidelines on the Identification and Treatment of Overweight and Obesity in Adults.* National Heart, Lung, and Blood Institutes. June 1998.

For adults, the concept of ideal body weight is taken from the life insurance industry's actuarial tables, which describe the weights of adult men and women associated with the lowest death rates. Table 4.1 shows the range of healthy body weights for adults, which are based on a person's height. If you are overweight, you will want to reduce until you're in the healthy range. For example, a woman who is five feet tall (60 inches) should aim at weighing 95 to

127 pounds. If she weighs 155 pounds, she is overweight. Table 7.2 (see page 103) shows the number of calories normal adults and overweight children should eat per day. To lose weight, this woman needs to eat no more than 1,600 calories per day. She also needs to exercise. At this calorie level, she should lose about half a pound to one pound per week, or one and a half to two pounds per week if she's exercising. Obviously, she'll lose weight faster with increased activity. Note: You do not want to lose more than two pounds per week, unless you are excessively obese and your doctor has approved accelerated weight loss.

However, the issues are different for children. Ideal body weight for children is more difficult to assess. The best data that we have for children shows that the normal body weight gives a BMI between the 5th and 85th percentiles. To estimate the ideal body weight for children 42 to 48 inches tall, allow one pound for each inch of their height. For children between 49 and 64 inches tall, add 4½ pounds for each inch above 48 inches.

For children, the need for calories is greater than for adults because they are growing. Younger children in particular need extra calories to expend as heat. This is especially true for newborns, who lose heat faster than adults, due to their greater surface area to body mass ratio. Newborns need about 60 calories per pound per day, a number that drops to about 20 to 30 calories per pound by mid-childhood.

For children in the normal range for weight, the rule of thumb for estimating calorie requirements and basic energy needs is 1,000 calories + 100 calories per year of age. This allows for normal amounts of exercise and permits additional calories for normal growth. For those children who are overweight, the problem is complicated if they are taller than average, exercise too little, and are more physically mature than normal for their age. For these children, it is better to estimate their calorie requirements based on their age (see Table 7.2 on page 103).

The Test

Before beginning the KidShape program, you will take a fitness test, adapted from the President's Council on Physical Fitness and Sports Challenge test. If this is the first time that you've exerted yourself after a prolonged period of inactivity, stretch gently but thoroughly before taking the test, using the stretches in Chapter 13. You will want to wear gym clothes and sneakers. Unless you are lucky enough to have a big yard with lots of gym equipment, you should plan to do this test in two stages. The first stage should be done at home and consists of curl-ups, push-ups, and V-sit reaches. The second stage should be done at a park or school playground with pull-up bars and, if possible, a running track, football field, or basketball court; this stage consists of an endurance walk/run, pull-ups, and a shuttle run.

This test is not for children under age six, who are still developing their locomotive skills and simply need time to practice running, jumping, skipping, hopping and tumbling. Forcing children under six to exercise can turn them off to physical activity over the long haul. Fortunately, most kids under six don't have to be prompted to be active and are welcome to join in the family exercises, moving, of course, at their own speed. For evaluative purposes, a BMI will suffice for younger children.

"KidShape is a program that kids will always carry within themselves. Once they learn, they can't go back to being ignorant or naïve."

—KidShape parent

Write down your test scores on the Information Survey form, and keep it in your folder or notebook, because you'll want to compare them to later scores. Remember that the purpose of this test is to evaluate your fitness levels, and not to compete against each other. The only person you're competing against is yourself. You may take the test as often as you like, or once you've finished all the workshops, or once every two months—whatever suits your schedule. Kids needn't worry about how they compare to their siblings, or to the peers and classmates at school. Your goal should be to always do better than the last time you took the test.

Allow time between events for participants to recover. You may drink water during the test, more on warm days than you might on cooler days, but don't drink so much that it sloshes around in your stomach.

TO BE DONE AT HOME
Part 1: Curl-ups

Lie on the floor with your knees bent and your feet about 12 inches from your buttocks. If you're uncomfortable, you may want to lie on a cushioned surface, thick carpeting, or a camping sleep pad, as long as the surface below you is firm. A bed, for instance, won't do.

Cross your arms and place your hands on your opposite shoulders. Have a partner hold your feet. Hold your elbows close against your chest and raise your trunk up until your elbows touch your thighs. Lie back down until your shoulders touch the floor. You have just completed one curl-up.

See how many curl-ups you can do in 60 seconds and record the number. Your partner should count out loud as you do them. These full curl-ups are recommended only for testing purposes and should not be part of your regular exercise regimen.

If you don't want to do full curl-ups because they put stress on the lower back, you can do modified curl-ups instead. You do not have to do both. Lie on your back as described, knees bent. This time, extend your arms forward with your fingers resting on your legs and pointed toward your knees. Your partner should cup his or her hands beneath your head. Curl your torso forward and slide your hands up your legs until your fingers touch your knees. Come back down until your head rests in your partner's hands again. That's a modified curl-up. Do as many as you can, with your partner counting "One thousand one, one thousand two, one thousand three," until you can't do any more at that pace. You can do modified curl-ups as part of your regular exercise.

Part 2: Push-ups

Lie on the floor face down with your hands under your shoulders, fingers straight and pointing forward, legs straight and slightly apart, toes to the floor. Push up with your arms until your arms are straight while keeping your back straight and your knees locked. Lower your body until you've made a 90-degree angle at the elbows (you do not have to bring your chin all the way down to the floor). See how many of these you can do in 60 seconds. Record the number. You can, if you wish, do bent-knee push-ups from a kneeling position.

Part 3: V-Sit Reach

This test measures your flexibility. Take your shoes off and sit on the floor with your legs extended in front of you. Your feet should be 8 to 12 inches apart, with your heels touching a line marked on the floor. This is the baseline. Take a ruler and place it on the floor between your feet, perpendicular to the baseline, which should bisect the ruler at the six-inch mark. Reach your hands out together in front of you, palms down, while your partner holds your legs straight. Point your toes up. Exhale as you reach forward as far as you can reach. Reach forward three times for practice, and then use the ruler to record how far forward you can reach on your fourth try.

TO BE DONE AT A PARK OR SCHOOL PLAYGROUND
Part 4: Endurance Walk/Run

At the timer's signal of "Ready, set—go!" you will all begin an endurance run on a safe marked course, such as the local high school track. It's okay to walk during the test, but you should try to complete the distance in the shortest time possible. Children six to seven years should do one lap, which is one quarter of a mile. Children eight to nine years should do two laps, one-half of a mile. Record your times.

Part 5: Pull-ups

Using either an overhand or an underhand grip, whichever is most comfortable, hang from a bar high enough that your feet don't touch the floor. Adults may need to give kids a boost so they can reach the bar. Kids need adults for spotters. Raise your body until your chin clears the bar, then lower yourself down to the starting position. Complete as many pull-ups as you can. Record the number. There is no time limit.

Part 6: Shuttle Run

Start with two lines about 10 yards apart. A good place to do the shuttle run is a football field with marked lines or a basketball court. The lines needn't be exactly 10 yards apart, as long as you use the same lines every time you take the test.

Place two objects behind one line, something you can reach down and pick up easily, such as small blocks of wood. Return to the opposite line and at the starting signal ("Ready, Set—Go!"), with someone timing you, run as fast as you can to the second line, pick up one block, run back to the first line and place the block on the floor behind the line. Do not throw or drop the blocks. After placing the first block, run back to the second line, pick up the second block and race back across the starting line. You don't have to place the second block down—the clock stops when you recross the starting line. Record your time.

WHAT PARENTS SHOULD KNOW

Ask your pediatrician about how much your overweight child should lose and how fast, or whether it's better to merely stop or slow weight gain, particularly if your child's BMI is above the 95th percentile. This will depend on the severity of the weight problem, how long your child has been overweight, and if the weight has caused other health problems.

Obesity is especially dangerous for young children. A two-year-old who weighs 65 pounds may have trouble walking or develop lower-leg fractures. Obesity in a six-year-old may contribute to asthma or obstructive sleep apnea. Obese teenagers may develop type 2 diabetes, high blood pressure, and high cholesterol. Obese children may also start puberty early, as young as seven or eight.

Once into puberty, girls' estrogens favor the laying down of fat, giving girls a higher percentage of body fat after puberty than boys. The high levels of testosterone that boys experience during puberty contribute to the rapid growth of muscle tissue, which burns calories fairly rapidly. With more muscle mass, adolescent boys tend to be somewhat less susceptible to obesity than girls.

CHAPTER 5

WORKSHOP 1
Establishing the Basics

This first workshop will introduce you and your family to the basic components of the program. You'll learn about different food groups and the food guide pyramid, and develop an activities pyramid as well. You will also learn how to support each other through active listening.

You may again want to have one of the grown-ups serve as the team leader, at least at first, but bear in mind that the more your kids feel included in the decision-making, the more empowered they'll feel and the more motivated they'll become. They shouldn't feel like they're being forced to do something against their will, and they probably won't like to be told what to do. They should feel like equal partners. The leader may want to remind the team that this is a learning experience for everyone, and that you're all beginning a new experience.

At the First Meeting you talked about the point-rewards system. You should all begin by taking out your Weekly Point Charts (page 222) from your folders and rewarding yourself 10 points for attending Workshop 1. The leader should then tally the numbers from everyone's Weekly Point Charts on the Family Reward

Chart (page 223). At the next workshop, everyone will have many more points to add up, as you'll be receiving points for things you did the preceding week.

Then take turns reading aloud from the following Food for Thought section. Everyone should read one or two paragraphs before passing the book to the next person. Keep reading until you get to the "stop" sign that marks the end of the section (see page 57). Parents should, of course, help kids who are too young to read and explain the words that kids don't understand. Anyone who prefers to sit and listen without taking part in the reading is allowed to, but reading is encouraged—it's the best way to make sure everyone is involved and hearing what needs to be heard.

The Best Team You'll Ever Have Is Your Family

"Guess what?" Lucy Rodriguez told her mother Grace with great excitement. "I made the volleyball team!"

This was amazing news that only a few years earlier would have seemed utterly improbable, if not impossible. It was not that Grace doubted her daughter's determination or commitment, but only that the problem had existed for so long, and the task seemed so difficult.

Lucy had been a big baby, nearly 10 pounds at birth. At no point in her early childhood could Lucy have been considered thin. Being heavy was just a fact of life, Lucy thought, something she'd accepted and grown accustomed to, until high school. For most kids, high school is the biggest transition they have faced, and when they strongly want to fit in and be accepted. At age 15, Lucy was five feet four inches, 221 pounds, and extremely self-conscious about her size, worried what the kids at her new school were going to say.

After a visit to the doctor's office, a blood workup showed she had high blood pressure and elevated blood cholesterol. Her BMI was 38, hovering between obese and extremely obese for adults and well into the extreme range for children. But on the plus side, she was willing to work and sincerely committed to getting healthier.

Her parents committed the time to work with her. Grace and her husband, Ramon, made the time to prepare healthier foods instead of eating out in restau-

rants and fast-food places, and they exercised with Lucy, sometimes one or the other and sometimes both, depending on their schedules. It wasn't always easy because both Grace and Ramon worked, but Lucy appreciated the efforts they were making to help her and didn't want to let them down. At the same time, it was clear that she was doing this for herself, and not to please others.

After only three months of eating carefully and exercising, Lucy's weight was down to 198. Her first year of school was difficult, but the fact that she felt headed in the right direction made it easier for her. Knowing she was actively doing something made her feel more empowered, and that sense of empowerment carried over into other areas of her life. Because she knew that both her parents were helping her, she found it easier to talk about what was going on at school at the dinner table, while before she might have kept things to herself.

Eventually the exercise she was doing with her family wasn't enough. She heard about a summer program her school was offering, a volleyball "boot camp" requiring four-hour-long practices four times a week. To her parents, it sounded like a demanding schedule even for kids who were in shape, but Lucy wanted to do it. Sometimes she felt so tired at the end of the day that she wanted to quit, but with her parents' encouragement, she gutted it out. By the end of camp, her coach suggested she try out for the team in the fall. The morning of the tryouts, Grace and Ramon wished her luck, knowing she wouldn't want them to come watch, but Lucy knew they were at her side all the same.

"Can you believe it?" she said when she told her parents she made the team. She was proud to think of herself as an athlete for the first time in her life. "Our first game is Friday!"

At last report, Lucy weighed 178 pounds and is maintaining her weight. She continues to lead a healthier life.

Lucy's story illustrates how important it is for a child struggling with a weight problem to be supported by his or her family. Knowing they were there to help her eat right and exercise made all the difference.

It can make a difference in our family too.

Not all that long ago face-to-face conversation was the best entertainment a person could have. Families stayed involved in each other's daily lives, frequently through dinner table conversations. Kids reported on their days at school, or answered questions their parents asked about their homework or their social lives; current events, political or philosophical issues might be discussed; people might argue or discuss what they were going to wear to the prom—the subject didn't matter. What was important was that families talked together.

Families still have conversations today, but for many people, they are infrequent and too brief. Think of how busy our lives seem these days. With computers and personal digital assistants, cordless phones, cell phones, Internet, newspapers, magazines, cable television, radio, VCRs, and DVDs, we have a million things that distract us from each other and a million things to do other than talk to each other.

In a way, a level of intimacy has been lost that was once taken for granted. Even something like eating dinner with the television on adds a layer of clutter to our conversation, a background of noise that fills in the silences. Times have changed, but we *can* create a space in family life for conversation.

Effective communication takes time and patience, both scarce in busy families. Time is a major barrier, particularly for families where both parents work outside the home, and kids are busy with school, friends, and other activities. Getting fit together as a family will involve a commitment of time, but it is time that will benefit all of us. Getting everyone on the same schedule may require all of us to shift our priorities somewhat. We need to remember that the actions we're taking can create health benefits that will last a lifetime—what could be more important than that?

The key is to simply meet at the breakfast, lunch, or dinner table at specific times, as often as possible, without a television, radio, CD, or computer on. Handheld computer games and reading materials should be left in another room, and if the phone rings, we will let the answering machine pick it up.

Then we will talk.

We need to talk honestly about being overweight without risking hurt feelings or making anyone feel defensive. Parents should speak in a way that's loving, supportive, and constructive. Kids should be able to speak knowing they're not going to be blamed. The goal is to understand the complexities of the problem. Once we begin to understand all the causes for obesity—including high-calorie sugars and highly saturated fats, bigger serving sizes, and our increasingly inactive lifestyle—becoming overweight really does start to seem like something no single person can take all the blame for.

As with any team, it's counterproductive when members start criticizing or blaming each other. In professional sports, teams at the bottom of the standings may resemble a family in trouble, with some players not speaking to their teammates, or badmouthing or blaming them. The teams on top have players who have faith in each other and encourage each other. Team members can defeat their own self-doubt simply by saying, "I may not believe in myself, but my teammates believe in me." It's amazing what we can accomplish when we keep our self-doubts in check. This is true in sports and in business—and in our family as well.

Remember that no one became overweight overnight. It's going to take time to see results. We should have realistic goals and expectations. The changes we need to make may seem overwhelming: limiting our time in front of the TV, cooking dinner at home more often, buying healthier foods, and exercising every day. If we tried to make all of these changes at once, we *would* be overwhelmed. But if we take a number of small steps, we can master these one at a time. Setting reasonable and achievable goals will pay off, and the successful feeling we get reaching one goal empowers us to try the next one.

What's difficult is that we are altering the things that give us comfort—such as the familiar foods we have been eating, and our TV habits. This is going to require diligent effort. It may, for a while, be uncomfortable. Sometimes we may not see the results we might hope to see right away, and we may get discouraged. That's where it's to our advantage to be part of a team—if one person starts to feel overwhelmed or as if what we're doing is too difficult, someone else is there to give a hand. And no one has to carry the whole load.

In the end, everyone should remember and say to himself or herself: "I can do more as a member of a team than I could ever do alone, and the best team I'll ever have is my family."

STOP

Check-in

When you're finished reading, the team leader should ask for reactions or feelings about what's just been read. It's important that everybody understands that you can all speak freely about whatever is on your mind. This is the time and the place to practice active listening, as described on pages 59–60. In the first workshop, you should share how things are going for you, your hopes for the program, your goals, and your fears or chief concerns.

If people are hesitant to speak or don't know what to say, the leader may ask the following questions. Parents as well as kids should try to answer them.

1. What does it mean for you to be starting the program?

2. What goals are you hoping to achieve?

3. How can we help each other achieve those goals?

4. What things do you think caused your weight gain?

5. How do you feel at mealtime when the whole family eats together? Peaceful or stressed? Hectic or relaxed?

6. Think of the last three times a friend or family member offered to help you—how did you feel? Were they able to understand your feelings?

7. Is it easier when a family member is involved in your weight loss program, or do they annoy or pressure you and make it harder?

8. What kind of support would you most appreciate?

9. Name four people, besides your parents, whom you can trust with your problems.

10. What are the biggest obstacles you'll need to overcome to lose weight?

Now each family member should fill in Your Personal Food and Fitness Survey (page 231), which should be in everyone's folder. Answer the questions about your eating and activities honestly, and keep the survey in your folder. You will take this survey again when you have completed the workshops, and be able to compare your answers before and after the program.

Learning to Really Listen

The most critical component of effective communication is what therapists call "active listening"—when you confirm and validate what someone has said. Often when someone is talking to us, our attention drifts off. We start to think of something we're reminded of, or begin to formulate what we're going to say before the other person is finished speaking. Just as often, we only hear what we want to hear, or we only listen for as long as it takes us to think we know the gist of what the other person is saying. And sometimes the person speaking hasn't said exactly what they're trying to say, or has misspoken in a way that's confusing or misleading.

Active listening is used in a variety of therapies to help people having communication problems, though it works just as well where the goals are more general. It's similar to the way psychotherapists listen to their patients, and though it sounds easy, it's more difficult than it seems and takes time to perfect. Simply put, active listening is a four-part process.

PART 1. First, the speaker is given an opportunity to speak without being interrupted. That alone can be a breakthrough, as too often we interrupt and cut each other off. During the first phase, the listener notes what the speaker is saying without drifting off or formulating responses, with the understanding that the listener will get a chance to speak also.

PART 2. The listener recites back to the speaker what they've heard and asks if they got anything wrong or left anything out. It is sometimes surprisingly difficult to say back the things we've heard accurately, but it gets easier with practice.

PART 3. The speaker answers the question, correcting what the listener got wrong or reemphasizing points the listener omitted.

PART 4. The listener validates what the speaker has said by making a statement of empathy that expresses understanding. This is not a time to say "I know how I'd feel if that happened to me," which is a common response, but rather it's a time to see through another person's eyes. You need to feel what *they* might feel, from *their* perspective, which is the difference between empathy and sympathy. It's a time for comfort, not confrontation. Even if you think they are wrong, you need to understand how they could reach the conclusions they've reached and let them know that they're justified and entitled to their feelings, regardless of your interpretation. For example, if your child complains that all the other kids at school get to eat Skittles or M&Ms, your response might be, "Yes, I can see how unfair that feels. What do you think about those choices that your friends are making? Are they good choices or bad ones?"

Activity 1: Introducing the Food Pyramid

The typical home food environment that can lead to obesity includes a lot of foods high in fat and in sugar. Usually meals are not planned, allowing family members to acquire most of their calories from snacks, sweets, crackers, cookies, and other high-calorie foods with low nutritional value. Family members also frequently eat meals outside the home, which are generally high in fat, calories, and sodium, and rarely include fruits and vegetables.

Now look at Figure 5.1. Developed by KidShape dietitians, the KidShape food guide pyramid depicts the relative amounts you should eat from the basic food groups. It is designed especially for families trying to manage their weight and is slightly different from the USDA's food guide pyramid. The KidShape food guide pyramid places starchy vegetables, such as potatoes, corn, and peas, in the grain group. The dairy group contains only milk and yogurt. Cheese is placed in the protein group as a high-fat protein, and ice cream is placed in the fats and sweets category.

The food guide pyramid is especially useful because it provides a tool for looking at diets from a variety of ethnic groups or cultures (see Table 5.1). This means that people from diverse backgrounds can use it to plan balanced meals. It also means that it can help you choose a balanced meal at a Mexican restaurant or at a

Chinese restaurant. While the vegetables may be different in appearance and taste, the constant is the serving size. The same can be said for items in each of the various groups. The key to successfully navigating through different ethnic foods is to correctly identify the food group to which each item belongs. Then it is simple, if you understand the food guide pyramid, to construct a balanced meal.

The message to be taken from the food guide pyramid is that we should eat a variety of foods from all of the food groups each day. Look at the bottom tier of the pyramid, the group for grains. From the shape of the pyramid, it is obvious that foods from the grain group should provide the foundation of our diet and provide us with the majority of our daily calories. A grain is generally a plant seed, most often from the grass family, and it supplies us with the carbohydrates we need.

In the grain group are complex carbohydrates, including whole grain breads, brown rice, and whole grain cereals. Other foods that are complex carbohydrates, and that are also on this level of the pyramid, are starchy vegetables such as potatoes, corn, and peas. Complex carbohydrates take time to be digested and do not cause a quick rise in blood sugar. Many contain fibers that help to limit the absorption of fats and cholesterol. They also are good sources of essential vitamins and minerals. You should have from 6 to 11 servings of complex carbohydrates per day, depending on your age and weight.

Use a copy of the blank pyramid on page 232 (it should be in each participant's folder) or draw one on a piece of paper. Now, in the bottom tier, write down all the grain-based foods you can think of.

The next food groups are vegetables and fruit, which are both on the second level of the pyramid. These groups include food such as lettuce, broccoli, and carrots for vegetables, and apples, oranges, and bananas for fruit. Generally it's better to choose whole, fresh fruits, which are rich in vitamins and fibers. You should count only 100 percent fruit juice as one fruit serving, and limit juice to only one of your fruit servings per day. Fruit "drinks" contain mostly sugar and very little actual fruit. You can use canned fruit, but look at the labels to be certain that it is fruit packed in its own juice, without extra sugar. You should have 2 to 4 servings of fruit per day. Along with fruits, vegetables are high in fiber and low in fat and sodium. They provide a range of important nutrients. Green leafy vegetables are high in beta-carotene, vitamin C, calcium, and iron, whereas yellow vegetables such as squash are high in vitamin A. Some dietitians recommend

KIDSHAPE
FOOD GUIDE PYRAMID

FIGURE 5.1

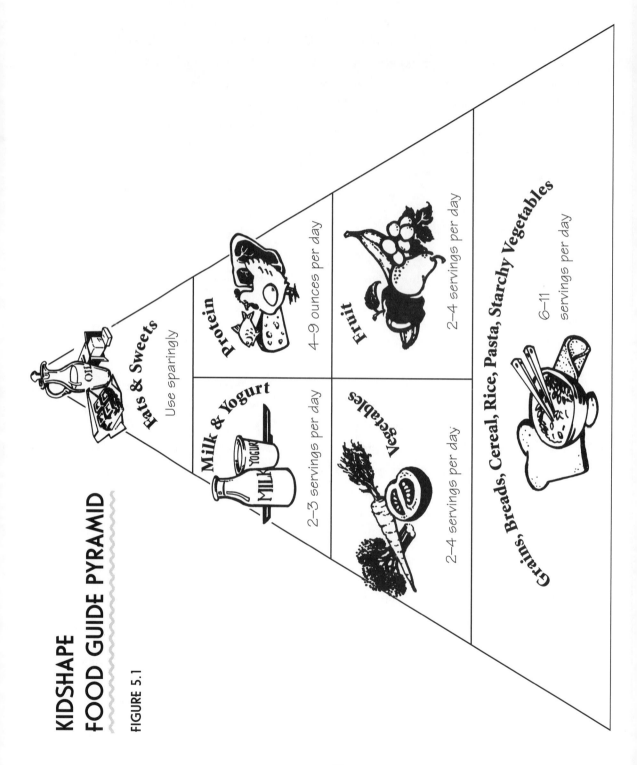

Fats & Sweets
Use sparingly

Protein
4–9 ounces per day

Fruit
2–4 servings per day

Milk & Yogurt
2–3 servings per day

Vegetables
2–4 servings per day

Grains, Breads, Cereal, Rice, Pasta, Starchy Vegetables
6–11 servings per day

FOOD GROUPS FROM THE FOOD GUIDE PYRAMID

Table 5.1

Food group	Sample foods with portion sizes	Latino foods	Southern foods	Asian foods	Indian foods	Jewish foods	Mediterranean foods
Grains 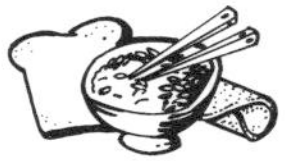	1 slice whole wheat bread ½ hot dog/hamburger bun ¾ c. unsweetened cereal ½ c. cooked cereal 6 saltine-type crackers ½ c. cooked noodles/rice ½ c. mashed potatoes ½ c. corn or peas	1 small corn tortilla ½ flour tortilla ½ c. posole ½ c. rice ½ c. corn	½ c. grits, cooked ½ c. sweet potatoes, yams ½ c. rice ½ c. macaroni noodles 1 square corn bread ½ c. corn or peas	½ c. rice ½ c. glutinous (sticky) rice ½ c. rice congee ½ c. noodles ½ c. vermicelli	1 small naan ½ c. rice (regular/ basmati/ jasmine) 1 small plantain	½ small bagel 1 matzo ½ c. kasha ½ c. bulgur 1 small slice challah	½ c. pasta ½ c. risotto ½ c. couscous ½ c. polenta ½ c. bulgur
Vegetables 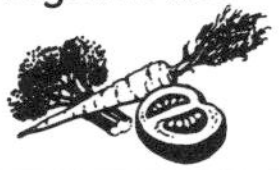	1 c. raw vegetables, like lettuce or tomatoes ½ c. cooked vegetables, like broccoli or carrots	Nopales Jicama Tomato Chayote	Okra Tomatoes Squash Greens	Bok choy Leeks Eggplant	Cucumber Mung bean sprouts Okra Eggplant	Borscht	Eggplant Spinach Artichoke Mushrooms
Fruit 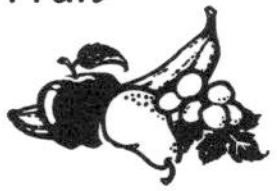	Small apple 16 grapes ½ (9-inch) banana ½ c. 100% fruit juice (limit juice to ½ c. per day)	1 zapote ½ mango ½ papaya 1 small plantain	Fresh fruit	1 kumquat ½ mango 1 guava 2–3 ditchi or lychee ½ persimmon	½ mango 1 guava	Fresh fruit	2 dried figs ½ c. raspberries ½ grapefruit
Milk & Yogurt 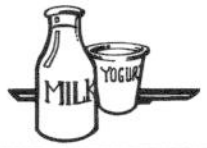	1 c. 1% low-fat or nonfat milk 1 c. 1% low-fat or nonfat yogurt	1 c. milk	1 c. milk 1 c. low-lactose or lactose-free milk 1 c. buttermilk	1 c. milk	1 c. lassi (blended nonfat yogurt)	1 c. milk	1 c. milk 1 c. yogurt
Protein 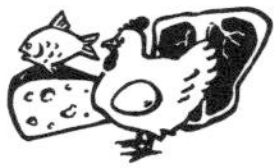	1 oz. lean protein, like chicken/ turkey without skin, lean beef/pork/lunch meats, fresh fish, tuna packed in water ½ c. beans/lentils/soybean products 1 egg or 2 egg whites 2 Tbsp. natural sugar-free peanut butter ½ to ¾ c. low-fat or nonfat cottage cheese	Chicken Beef Chorizo (with fat drained) Beans Queso blanco Queso asadero Queso cotija	Ham Chicken Red beans Black-eyed peas	Seafood Soybeans Tofu Beef	Chicken Garbanzo beans Other beans Paneer	Lox Whitefish Chicken Beef brisket Salmon Chickpeas Lentils	Fish Lean beef/veal Beans/lentils Ricotta cheese Mozzarella cheese
Fats & Sweets 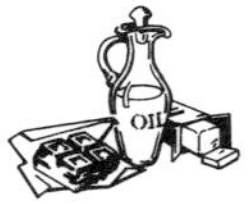	2 small cookies ½ c. ice cream 1 tsp. butter, margarine, mayonnaise 1 Tbsp. reduced-fat salad dressing	1 tsp. lard 1 tsp. butter 1 small piece candy 1 tsp. crema	½ oz. fatback	1 Tbsp. coconut milk	1 tsp. ghee 1 tsp. cooking oil	1 tsp. cream cheese 1 tsp. tahini	1 tsp. olive oil 1 tsp. butter 1 tsp. pine nuts 1 tsp. tahini

eating by color, meaning that you select vegetables that are yellow, green, red, purple, and white, in order to assure that you get the full range of nutrients. You should have 2 to 4 servings of vegetables per day.

Using your blank food pyramid, in the second tier write down all the vegetables and fruits you can think of.

The last two food groups are dairy and protein, which are also important for a well-balanced diet and come mainly from animals. The dairy group includes milk and yogurt. It is the main dietary source of calcium, which is needed at all ages. We all know that calcium is important for building strong bones and teeth in growing children, but it's equally important in maintaining the bones of adults. When bones weaken and lose their density, osteoporosis is the result. Dairy foods also provide protein, B vitamins, and vitamin D. You should consume 2 to 3 servings of milk or yogurt per day. The protein group includes beef, pork, chicken, fish, nuts, beans, lentils, and soybeans. Because dairy and protein contain more calories, they take up less space on the pyramid, which means you don't need to eat as much of these food groups as you do the fruits, vegetables, and grains at the base of the pyramid.

On the third tier of your blank pyramid, write down all the different kinds of dairy products and proteins you can think of.

At the tip of the pyramid are fats, oils, and sugars—foods that contain the most energy of all the food groups. Fat *is* an essential nutrient, so we do need some, but most of us eat far too much for our health. If you were working as a lumberjack or driving a dogsled and burning several thousand calories a day, you could probably eat a fair amount of fats, oils, and sugars and not gain weight. But few of us live at such a sustained activity level, so most of us need to eat only sparingly from the food group at the top of the pyramid. It is important to limit fat intake, but as you can see from Table 7.2 (page 103), a certain amount of fat is allowed each day. In fact, the food guide pyramid is based on the understanding that 30 percent of an individual's calories will come from fat. We say to eat fat "sparingly" because some foods, especially those prepared commercially, have a much higher amount of fat than a similar item prepared at home. Thus, the amount of fat in your diet might not be easy to estimate.

On the top of your pyramid, everybody write down all the different kinds of fats, oils, and sweets you can think of. Include fats and sugars you eat combined in a single product, such as a cookie or cracker.

You ran out of space in the pyramid to write down all the foods you could think of in this last group, didn't you? What do you think that means?

Now take a look at the Weekly Food Log, which should be in each participant's folder (see pages 216–217). To complete the food log, each person should write down the name and amount of each food eaten, as well as the date and time it was eaten. If you eat more than one food at a meal or snack, put each food item on a separate line. For example, a sandwich, an apple, and a glass of milk at lunch go on three separate lines (the sandwich counts as one item). Include all drinks, except for water. In addition, use the numerical scale on the form to indicate how hungry you were when you started eating the meal or snack and when you finished. Use the scale to rate your hunger before and after each meal or snack as a whole—you do not need to rate each food item separately. Use the column on the right to write down any special feelings before and after eating. If you were bored, angry, upset, or experiencing some other feeling, write it down.

You should complete this log daily, using as many "continued" pages as you need, and review it as you proceed through the program. Completing the food log provides you with an opportunity to monitor yourself and to learn about the feelings that trigger eating behaviors associated with certain foods at certain times. Keeping a food log also allows you, as you learn more about nutrition, to see where certain changes need to be made.

Good and Not-So-Good Carbohydrates

Experts have been hotly debating whether or not grains deserve the dominant place they hold at the bottom of the food pyramid. Many opponents of the food pyramid claim its structure was an outcome of a power struggle between meat producers and grain growers, with the heavily subsidized grain industry winning out. Others suggest that the food pyramid, with its emphasis on carbohydrates, has actually contributed to the rise in obesity in the United States. They observe that the increase in obesity to its present epidemic proportions began around 1992, at the same time that the food guide pyramid was introduced. There may be some truth to this claim, and some experts speculate that the food guide pyramid is due for a major overhaul in the next year or so, and that at that time it is likely that the bottom of the pyramid will be fruits and vegetables, with grains listed above them. Despite this controversy, the concept of a diet that has as its base foods made of complex carbohydrates, such as whole wheat bread, brown rice, whole grains, and unprocessed or minimally processed fruits and vegetables, appeals to many clinical dietitians.

However, even dietitians who advocate carbohydrates agree that there are "good" and "bad" carbohydrates. "Bad" carbohydrates are thought to be those with what's called a high glycemic index. This means they break down quickly into sugars. They cause a spike in your blood sugar (glucose), which triggers a sudden release of large amounts of insulin, which then rushes the excess blood sugar into storage. High blood glucose also inhibits the function of a substance called glucagon, a hormone that directs the body to burn stored fuel reserves. Once blood sugar levels fall to normal or below, the body needs more energy, but because glucagon has been inhibited, the result is increased hunger an hour or two after eating. Bad carbohydrates are those found in refined flours, white bread, instant oatmeal, most potatoes, white rice, and regular pasta.

"Good" carbohydrates are made from whole grains that contain the grain's outer layer (or bran) and the inner germ. You will find whole grains in whole wheat bread, brown rice, couscous, buckwheat groats, millet, bulgur wheat, bran flakes, oat squares, and whole wheat pasta. Because whole grains are higher in fiber (a cup of whole wheat flour has 14.5 grams of fiber per cup, compared to 3.4 grams in refined white bleached flour, reports an article in *Pediatrics*), they digest more slowly and have a lower glycemic index. This, in turn, results in more level blood sugar, and avoids the hunger that results from dips in your blood sugar.

Carbohydrates remain an important part of your diet, but you should eat whole grains rather than refined starches whenever possible.

Activity 2: Introducing the Activity Pyramid

Spend a few minutes talking about physical activity. What is it? What do you think it does for you?

Take a piece of paper and all of you brainstorm and write down all the reasons why physical activity might be good for you. (Possible answers: it's fun; it can be a stress reliever; it is a way to spend time together; it can help you manage your weight.)

Take a look at the KidShape family activity pyramid in Figure 5.2, which is set up much like the food guide pyramid. Sedentary activities such as watching television are at the top of the pyramid, and you will want to limit these activities, as you limit the fats and sweets at the top tier of the food pyramid. Activities that burn the most calories are at the bottom—you will want to do lots of these.

Take another piece of paper and write down all the things you do (or could do) during the day and then decide where they would fit into the various sections of the activity pyramid. One person should write the activities down while the others discuss where they should go.

In the same way that it's essential to keep a food log, it is also helpful to keep a record of your weekly activities. The key to good health and successful weight maintenance is daily exercise. Adults should get at least 30 minutes per day of moderate physical activity (something that makes you sweat and raises your heart rate). Children ages 6 to 16 need at least 60 minutes per day of moderate physical activity, some of which they may get in school. The best way to assure that both parents and children get enough physical activity is to start with 30 minutes at least three times per week. Each participant should have a Weekly Activity Log in his or her folder (see page 218). You should complete this form every day by putting a check in the box for each physical activity you did for at least 30 minutes.

KIDSHAPE
FAMILY ACTIVITY
PYRAMID

FIGURE 5.2

Source: Adapted with permission from *The Kid's Activity Pyramid* © 1996 Park Nicollet *HealthSource*, Park Nicollet Institute, Minneapolis, U.S.A., 1-800-372-7776.

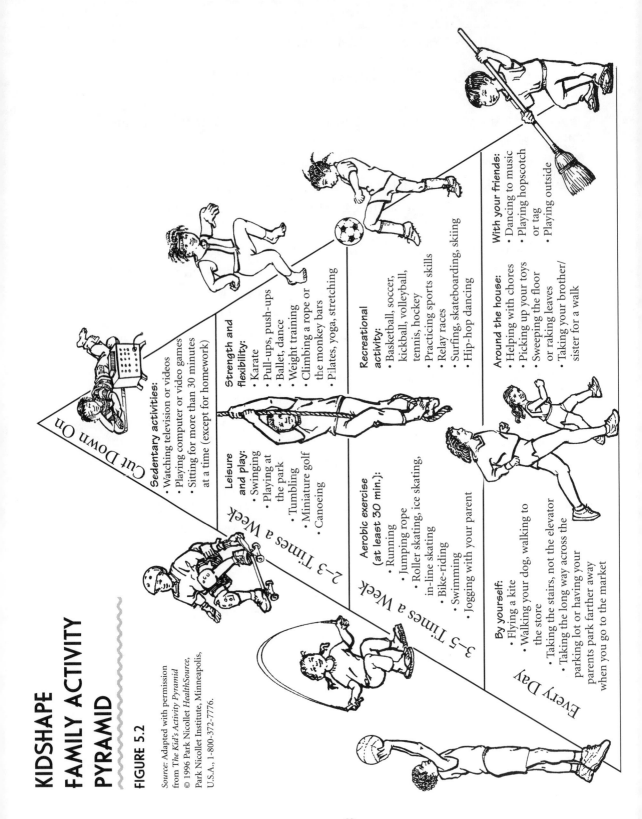

Cut Down On

Sedentary activities:
- Watching television or videos
- Playing computer or video games
- Sitting for more than 30 minutes at a time (except for homework)

2–3 Times a Week

Strength and flexibility:
- Karate
- Pull-ups, push-ups
- Ballet, dance
- Weight training
- Climbing a rope or the monkey bars
- Pilates, yoga, stretching

Leisure and play:
- Swinging
- Playing at the park
- Tumbling
- Miniature golf
- Canoeing

3–5 Times a Week

Recreational activity:
- Basketball, soccer, kickball, volleyball, tennis, hockey
- Practicing sports skills
- Relay races
- Surfing, skateboarding, skiing
- Hip-hop dancing

Aerobic exercise (at least 30 min.):
- Running
- Jumping rope
- Roller skating, ice skating, in-line skating
- Bike-riding
- Swimming
- Jogging with your parent

Every Day

With your friends:
- Dancing to music
- Playing hopscotch or tag
- Playing outside

Around the house:
- Helping with chores
- Picking up your toys
- Sweeping the floor or raking leaves
- Taking your brother/sister for a walk

By yourself:
- Flying a kite
- Walking your dog, walking to the store
- Taking the stairs, not the elevator
- Taking the long way across the parking lot or having your parents park farther away when you go to the market

Activity 3: Writing Attainable Goals

It's important to have goals. A goal puts what you want to have happen into words. The best goals are specific, measurable, and attainable. What is an attainable goal? It can be measured, and it's small enough that you can do it easily. If your goal is something like, "I will eat more sensibly," that's too vague. If your goal is something like, "I will eat four servings of fruit every day," then you can keep track and know how many days you've achieved these goals. The goal, "I will lose 15 pounds" is measurable, but it's too large a goal to achieve in a short time period. "I will get more exercise" is too vague. "I will play one-on-one basketball with Dad twice this week" is specific, measurable, achievable, and fun.

"KidShape focuses on good health— not necessarily on weight loss. It was valuable for parents and children to share."

—KidShape parent

Writing down a goal is the first step to accomplishing it. Think of things you can change about the way you eat and live. Can you take the stairs instead of the elevator? That's a small attainable goal that will, in the long term, lead to greater health.

Each family member should have a Weekly Goals form (see page 219) and a supply of stickers in his or her folder. (Participants, especially adults, may elect not to use stickers.) As part of each workshop, you will be given two goals related to eating, and two goals related to physical activity, which you will write down on your Weekly Goals form. During the week, you will put a sticker in the goal-tracking boxes at the bottom of the form for every day you met your goals. You will then have a record of your goals and your progress toward meeting them. Your goals for this week are the following:

1. I will eat a healthy breakfast.

2. I will eat two fruits in one day.

3. I will stretch for 10 minutes (see pages 170–176).

4. I will limit TV viewing to less than two hours in one day.

Physical Activity

At the end of your first workshop, make a schedule that everyone can agree on to meet and exercise at least three times during the week. Using the activity pyramid as a guideline, discuss what specific physical activities you each like to do. Turn to the lists of activities in Chapter 12 to get additional ideas. The family can then plan out activities to do together, ranging from exercises such as walking or running to more unusual activities such as hula hoops, salsa dancing, kick boxing, treasure hunting, or running an obstacle course that you can build in the backyard.

If you have time, do one session now, when everyone is already together: Everyone should stretch for 10 minutes and then exercise for 30 minutes, choosing one or more stretches from Chapter 13 and an activity from Chapter 12. Be sure to start "slow and easy," especially if some of you aren't used to exercise, and choose activities that are fun for everybody. Anyone who feels extreme discomfort or pain should back off.

Keeping a Journal

Everyone should keep a journal. You can use the Weekly Journal Page (Child or Adult), which should be in your folder (see pages 220–221). The simplest way to start keeping a journal, and the way that often works best with younger children, is to use the numerical scale on the Weekly Journal Page to answer the questions related to eating and exercise. A good place to note positive points in the day is in the space labeled "Name one good thing that happened today." Finally, using the space designated "My thoughts," you can try to answer some of the following questions.

1. Am I trying to do too many things at once?

2. Am I letting my family help me?

3. Am I listening? Am I truly understanding and supporting my loved ones?

4. Am I paying attention to what I eat and what my activities are?

5. Am I committed to sticking with the program?

6. What do I hope to gain from the program?

7. What are my short-term goals?

8. What are my long-term goals?

The personal journal provides a way for you to become more aware of your feelings toward exercise and other daily activities. It also provides a space where you can focus on the positive aspects of your life. You should complete an entry each day of the week. These are private pages. You can share items from them with others if you want to, but you don't need to. Just let your team leader see that you have completed at least four days per week in order to get reward points.

For those who wish to write more, particularly older children or parents, this may be an opportunity to begin the rewarding activity of journal keeping. If you are so inclined, you may want to buy a blank spiral notebook or composition book and write more extensive answers to these questions (if you are already using a binder, you can just add blank paper to it).

Homework Assignment

To make the most effective use of your time, each workshop involves hands-on activity and some homework. The five tasks critical to your success are keeping track of what you eat, keeping track of and increasing your physical activity, goal setting, and keeping in touch with your feelings and moods. That's why, with each workshop, you will be asked to complete a Weekly Food Log, a Weekly Activity Log, Weekly Goals, and a Weekly Journal Page. These pages should be in each participant's folder and can be found on pages 216–221. Remember that completing these pages each week allows you to earn points toward the rewards that your team has set.

In addition to the weekly pages, each workshop has another homework assignment that helps you review what you learned or prepare for the next workshop. This workshop's assignment focuses on physical activity. Exactly what is it that you do every day? Do you know what your actual activity level is? Perhaps you're more active than you think you are, or perhaps less.

Take another look at the activity pyramid in Figure 5.2. Using your Weekly Activity Log, in which you are recording your physical activities during the week, draw another blank pyramid (or use a copy of the one on page 232) and make a mark in the various tiers for every session of your leisure time activities. (You can do this individually or as a family.)

Last but not least, be sure to fulfill the commitment you made in the contract to eat together as a family at least five times a week and to exercise together at least three times a week for 30 minutes.

WHAT PARENTS SHOULD KNOW

The more kids learn about the causes and reasons for obesity, the easier it is on those who feel like they're overweight because they're doing something wrong. They won't understand this by themselves. They have to be told and taught by someone who cares about them, preferably their primary role models—you.

Parents need to keep everyone involved and motivated. Workshops may be done with one parent and child, but the more family members who participate, the better. Usually everyone can benefit, and it's better for the overweight child not to be singled out. And if a child sees a parent or older sibling eating healthfully, she'll be far more likely to do it herself than if she's simply told to do it.

Sometimes one family member may be too busy, too stressed out, or too defensive to join in. That's okay. Often, as your weight, mood, and energy levels start to improve, other family members notice and ask to join in. Require that nonparticipating family members refrain from sabotaging others: If they want ice cream or potato chips, they must have those foods outside the home.

Remember that families don't operate like businesses. Family members respect, admire, love, and imitate each other and crave each other's approval. Children love their parents and, from the very youngest ages, want to be just like them and do what they do. It shouldn't surprise us when we see a child chow down just like Dad or want to join in when Mom takes an afternoon cookie break. And neither should it surprise us when kids imitate the good things we do.

CHAPTER 6

WORKSHOP 2

Deciding How Much to Eat

The primary goal of this workshop is to learn how to distinguish between how much food we truly need to eat, and how much we *feel* we need to eat, based on our own sense of what seems right.

Remember the point-rewards system that we talked about at the First Meeting? Now is the time for family members to add up the points they earned since the previous workshop on their Weekly Point Charts. The leader should then tally the numbers from everyone's Weekly Point Charts on the Family Reward Chart. Then, take a few minutes to discuss the previous workshop and activities, and if desired, share things from your Weekly Journal Pages. Make sure that everybody has a chance to say what's on his or her mind and that you practice "active listening" if one of your kids has something to say. Does anybody have any questions? How does everyone feel? Does anyone have any suggestions as to how things might be improved or made easier?

When you're done, take turns reading aloud from the following:

Using Food as a Substitute for Love

By the time Linda came to see her doctor, she'd gained 110 pounds in the previous 16 months, which had caused high blood pressure and mild diabetes. She was only 13 years old, a seventh grader, but weighed 271 pounds. To make things even tougher, Linda was starting over at a new school after moving with her mother, Sandra, from out of state.

It's difficult for any new kid in school, and worse for obese kids. Linda was finding it impossible to fit in at her new school. She had very few friends. The only attention she got was from the boys, who teased her with rude and suggestive comments. Such comments made Linda feel even more self-conscious, and Linda already felt extremely uncomfortable with her body, which had recently showed signs of the onset of puberty.

Her mother, Sandra, said that where they used to live Linda had friends to play with after school. In recent months, Linda would come home from school and immediately turn on the television, which she would watch for seven or eight hours at a stretch. Excessive television watching, psychologists know, is often a way children hide or mask depression.

"Is there anything Linda might be feeling sad about?" Sandra was asked.

"Well," Sandra said, "you know, she's had a hard life."

"How so?"

Sandra was hesitant to speak at first. "Well, her father and I got divorced when she was only five, and that was hard for her. He was pretty abusive. That was when we got divorced, and I got sole custody, but he kept fighting it in the courts until the judge said I had to let her visit him. That was when we moved out of state because we had to get away from him."

Linda had been mistreated by her father. Her problems were compounded by the boys who teased her at school. She was referred to a psychologist who works with abused children and adolescents and is slowly working through her problems. She is beginning to eat healthier and take care of herself, now that she understands that the problems caused by her father were not her fault.

Little wonder that Linda's enormous emotional distress was expressing itself through her eating. For Linda, food was a reliable comfort, something that felt good going down and seemed to fill up an empty place inside of her.

The connection between food and emotional well-being begins in infancy. A baby cries out until somebody picks him up and puts something in his mouth. The sense of comfort and support is immediate: A warm body, a mother's soothing voice, a father's voice, all convey a sense of safety and well-being. The child bonds to the parent through the feeding process. Food is the first thing we know.

Parents sometimes use food as a reward or inducement. They bargain by saying, "If you finish your peas, you can have dessert." Sometimes when a child does something noteworthy, parents reinforce it with a favorite food. On birthdays, kids are allowed to indulge themselves to their hearts' content. What better way to cheer up a kid who's feeling blue than to buy an ice cream cone or a candy bar?

Kids learn from this how to use food as a form of "self-medication" once they learn how to open the refrigerator door or have access to convenience stores or vending machines. Childhood is when we identify foods as comforting, rather than nourishing.

Think about what foods we consider "comfort foods." Odds are, they are foods from childhood that gave us pleasure or satisfaction. The man who turns to chocolate milk and grilled cheese sandwiches or the woman who eats ice cream straight from the tub when things go wrong learned to modify their feelings with food as kids. So they return to these familiar foods when they feel a need to feel special and loved.

Sometimes we even eat foods we know are unhealthy, thinking, "I don't care—I've had a hard day—I *deserve* this."

But why would we deserve to be rewarded with something bad for us?

The reality is that we can be nicer to ourselves and treat ourselves better by becoming informed about the ways we hurt ourselves with food. We shouldn't use food to make us feel better. We should feel good about ourselves, and then eat.

It is, of course, wonderful to enjoy the pleasure of eating good food in good company. There are even sensible ways to enjoy "comfort" foods, as long as we keep them in proper proportion. But there are more effective ways to comfort ourselves than eating. Sometimes the fastest way to make ourselves thin is to first make ourselves proud. We can and should feel proud of ourselves at every step of the journey, proud that we're moving in the right direction, and proud to be part of a winning team.

Overweight kids have a lot to overcome. Overweight kids are frequently traumatized in school, sometimes daily. They're called names. They may be laughed at in gym class, and chosen last for sports. They may get poked or squeezed or touched in other inappropriate ways. They often sit alone in the cafeteria, where they focus on their food, rather than looking around to see who might be laughing at them. Some overweight kids learn to make jokes at their own expense, calling attention to their own obesity before somebody else does.

All the hurt feelings and social isolation drive overweight children to turn to food for comfort, while pushing them toward passive, solitary pastimes. Too often, an overweight kid will stay indoors, reading books, watching television, or playing video games and consuming potato chips and soda while the kids he wishes were his friends play loudly outside.

Being overweight involves problems that won't simply disappear overnight when we begin to lose weight—though losing weight can be part of the solution. There is no time limit to reach our goals. The philosophy of eating healthy foods and exercising is not something to be picked up and put down once we're thinner, nor is it a crash plan to lose weight in the briefest amount of time. It a permanent change that will last a lifetime.

As we learn to make better choices about food and exercise and how to deal with people and difficult family situations, we will begin to feel more in control. It's important to give it time, and to continue to give support to each other. Even after we've finished the workshops, we will need to remember that the journey has just begun.

The difficulties associated with being overweight are heartbreaking, but the sooner we start addressing them, the better. We must separate emotions from eating behaviors now, when bad habits are easier to break. Breaking the vicious cycle occurs gradually, one step at a time. By working together as a family, we can greatly improve our physical health, and at the same time become happier, more confident, and more energized. By doing it together, we have someone to share the journey with. When a family promises to help each other eat and exercise sensibly, it's easier for everyone.

STOP

Check-in

Ask for reactions to what you've just read, again engaging in active listening. That's particularly important today, because emotional eating is often linked to kids feeling like they have no one to talk to. When parents seem judgmental, kids will hold back, saving the deeper subjects for their friends. A lot of eating comes when kids feel alone, often at the end of a cycle—the child wakes up in the morning, but the house is hectic with everyone rushing about to begin the day. School is full of classes, tests, questions from teachers, and comments from peers; then the child comes home, possibly to an empty house or one with preoccupied or busy parents, turns on the TV, opens a bag of chips, and disappears. An hour later, the chips are gone and the child is back in the kitchen, looking for something to eat. Kids use food to soothe themselves after a hard day—to calm themselves down and make themselves feel better and less empty. Food feels nurturing. It can be difficult for children to see how emotions and eating connect, or to understand that talking about their feelings is one of the best ways that they can feel better.

The team leader should ask family members:

1. How do you usually deal with your emotions?

2. When you have a bad day, at school or at work, what do you do during the day to make yourself feel better?

3. When you have a lousy day, what do you do when you come home? Is this a time when you eat more than usual?

4. If it is, are you eating because you're hungry? Or are you lonely or bored?

5. How do you feel after you have finished eating? Are you still lonely or bored?

6. When you get stressed or anxious, what do you do to calm yourself? If you eat, do you feel less nervous afterward?

7. Do you ever eat when you're sad? If you do, do you feel happier after a snack?

8. How do you feel inside when you feel lonely?

9. What kinds of situations make you feel like eating more than usual?

10. Is there a certain time of day that you tend to eat more?

When you've discussed these things and answered these questions, spend some time thinking about other things you could do to cheer yourself up besides eating. What are some activities or hobbies that may help you to feel better without resorting to food? You could try painting, riding a bicycle, walking the dog, visiting the library, or you could make plans to do something with a friend.

Activity 1: Developing a Buddy System

Sometimes kids turn to food when they feel they need help. But food won't listen to us, or comfort us, or tell us that it loves us. Yet sometimes we turn to food for support.

Instead, make a list of other people who can support you when you're having a rough time or a bad day. These can be friends, family, neighbors, teachers, or anybody whom you feel you can talk to. To help you do this, you should each answer the following questions (pertaining to your age group), taking a few minutes to talk it over, with parents helping the younger children. If kids would rather keep their thoughts private, they can write their answers on the back of their Weekly Journal Pages.

For children ages 6 to 10:

1. The last time you felt sad, whom did you go to or what did you do?

2. Is there someone who is good at making you feel better? If so, who is it?

3. When you last felt angry, could somebody help calm you down? If yes, who?

4. Who is a good person to go to for help when you are mad?

5. What do you do when you feel nervous?

Why We Turn to Comfort Foods

There may actually be a biological component to our "need" for comfort foods. A study on rats at the University of California in San Francisco seems to indicate that eating comfort foods counteracts the effects of the hormones we produce when we're under stress.

Stress is how the body reacts to perceived danger. A squirrel feels stress when a dog approaches. Humans feel stress when we look in the rearview mirror and realize someone is tailgating us, or when we're lying in bed wondering how we're going to pay the bills this month. In times of great danger, our adrenal gland produces adrenaline and other stress hormones to give us extra strength and responsiveness to protect ourselves. Stress hormones are also believed to interact with receptors in the brain to suppress appetite. Sometimes humans under great stress, such as those pacing in hospital emergency waiting rooms while a loved one is being operated on, forget to eat or don't feel hungry. In people who are under chronic stress, where several stressful things happen to them every day, their stress hormone levels stay elevated and they have a hard time feeling calm.

The UCSF study reported that rats with elevated stress hormone levels calmed down when fed high-energy foods. Among humans, comfort foods tend to be those with a high-energy and low-nutritional content—those loaded with fat or sugar or both.

While getting relief from comfort foods may make sense in a way, we all need to limit this type of eating and learn other ways to deal with stress. Remember that when you allow your lonely and unhappy child to overdose on television and comfort food or try to give emotional support by overfeeding your child, you compound the problem.

What names did you come up with? These people will be part of your support team, people you can go to for help when you're having a bad day. It's important to talk to people about your feelings—getting them out not only feels good, but can help you find a solution to problems. If you ask for help when you need it and share your feelings, you are guaranteed to feel better. If for some reason children and parents are uncomfortable discussing certain problems with each other, consider other people in your children's life who may be able to talk to them, including grandparents, aunts, uncles, teachers, neighbors, counselors, ministers, babysitters, or scout troop leaders.

Kids ages 11 or older, who may be more aware of their emotions, should answer the following questions:

1. Think about the last time a friend or family member offered to help you with a problem you were having—how did you feel?

2. Did they understand your feelings?

3. Is it easier when a buddy or family member tries to help you lose weight, or do they annoy or pressure you and make everything harder?

4. Has it ever seemed that you couldn't satisfy your hunger no matter how much you ate? How did you feel that day?

5. How do you deal with a bad day at school, a day when you failed a test or fought with a friend?

6. Do the ways your parents try to help you make you feel better or worse?

7. How could they best help you?

8. If you're uncomfortable getting help from them, who else could you turn to for support when you feel the need to talk? List three people whom you feel you could talk to or call on the telephone for support.

9. What else could you do, besides eat, if you're alone and feel like binging because of a bad day at school? Can you make a plan?

Questions for parents:

1. Do you believe your child is eating because of emotional stress?

2. Is your child able to talk to you, not just about shallow topics but about important things such as friends, relationships, problems, and fears?

3. Do you just guess at what your child is experiencing every day?

4. Do you know what may be causing anxiety or sadness in your child?

5. What after-school activities could you suggest or organize so that your child won't feel so alone?

6. Is there a new hobby or sport (active, not sedentary) that you could introduce to your child?

Activity 2: Portion Sizes

For this exercise, you will need measuring cups, measuring spoons, a food scale, plates, and bowls.

Last week, you learned about the basic food groups by working with the food guide pyramid. In each group, a certain number of servings were recommended—but what's a serving?

Recommended serving sizes are listed on the food labels that come attached to every food product you buy. We'll be talking in the next workshop about how many servings you will want to eat, but for now the goal is to familiarize yourselves with basic portions. The best way to do that is to practice measuring them.

Go to your cupboards or refrigerator and find 10 different food products, including liquids, with at least two food items from each food group in the pyramid.

Pour out the amount of each food that you usually eat. For example, if you're measuring cereal, fill a cereal bowl the way you ordinarily would. Try to guess how much that amount is in ounces, tablespoons, or cups. Do this for each of the foods you've taken from your cupboards.

Then look on the labels of each product. Take a measuring cup, a set of measuring spoons, or a food scale and measure out the exact recommended portion sizes. Put those portion sizes next to the amounts

"My son learned the importance of fat sources in food servings. Now he connects healthy eating and exercise with his long-term goals."

—KidShape parent

you usually eat. Is one portion bigger than the other? If so, which one is bigger? If not, congratulations—you've been eating the proper serving size.

Let the kids practice pouring out a half cup, a cup, two ounces, and so on, to help them become familiar with these amounts.

Now take out some bowls, cups, glasses, and plates that you ordinarily use. Using your measuring cups, measure out the standard serving sizes of foods and beverages such as cereal and orange juice, and transfer them to your dishes to see how they appear. This way, you will become familiar with what a real, day-to-day serving size should look like, and eventually you will not need to use the measuring cups.

Activity 3: Healthy Snacks

In your Weekly Food Log last week, you kept track of how hungry you were before and after you ate. Did you notice any patterns? How often did you feel like you were starving before you ate? Did you ever eat until you were beyond full?

We tend to overeat when we feel really hungry. The way to avoid feeling that hungry is to have healthy snacks between meals. Parent used to say, "Don't eat that—you'll ruin your appetite," but careful healthy snacking helps keep your appetite under control, and limits the amount of time you spend thinking about your next meal (and keeps you from feeling deprived). This doesn't mean it's okay to constantly graze all day long. The best plan is to have three healthy meals with one or two snacks in between.

Not just any snack will do either. Most snack foods appeal to our impulses and are sweet, fatty, and made with refined carbohydrates and other unhealthy ingredients. Can you think of snacks that are healthier?

You can choose from the list below. Remember to limit your portion to the serving size listed on the label or in Table 5.1. Note also that you should limit foods with artificial sweeteners to one or two servings per day.

HEALTHY SNACKS
→ Plain popcorn (air popped)
→ Low-fat or fat-free microwave popcorn

→ Rice cakes

→ Graham crackers

→ Gelatin (sugar free)

→ Fat-free pudding (consume in limited amounts)

→ Fat-free frozen bars (consume in limited amounts)

→ Fat-free frozen desserts (yogurt, ice cream, Italian ice cups; consume in limited amounts)

→ Angel food cake

→ Milkshake from skim milk and fat-free frozen yogurt or frozen dessert

→ Fresh fruit

→ Dried fruit

→ Applesauce

→ Raw vegetables with fat-free ranch dressing or nonfat sour cream dips

→ Unsweetened cereal, dry or with nonfat milk

→ Bagels with fat-free cream cheese

→ Pretzels

→ Fat-free potato or corn chips

→ Baked tortilla chips with bean dip or salsa

→ Fat-free saltines

→ Fat-free melba toast

→ Fat-free rye toast

→ Matzo

→ Low-fat quesadillas (fat-free cheese melted on non-lard, low-fat tortilla)

→ Low-fat cheese

→ Nonfat cottage cheese

→ Nonfat yogurt

→ Sugar-free sodas and drinks (consume in limited amounts)

Activity 4: Review Your Daily Activities

Now review your homework from last week. Participants should show their Weekly Food Logs and Weekly Activity Logs. Remember that while the intention is to make the progrom a positive experience, family members also can complain about part of the program or vent their frustrations.

For homework last week you prepared an activity pyramid based on your Weekly Activity Log. What does your activity pyramid look like? Do some sections have more marks in them than others? Are there sections that have none? As you review your activity pyramid for the past week, address the following questions:

1. How active have you been? Very? Not very? Moderately?

2. What activities do you do frequently?

3. What activities do you do infrequently?

4. Are there areas where you could improve?

5. What are two ways you could become more physically active?

Weekly Goals

On your Weekly Goals form, fill in the following goals:

1. I will use measuring cups to measure out correct portions of foods.

2. I will eat a healthy snack from the Healthy Snack list (pages 82–83).

3. I will try two new ways to be more physically active (_____ and _____).

4. I will spend time on my favorite hobby (_____).

Homework Assignment

Be sure to complete your Weekly Food Log, Weekly Activity Log, Weekly Goals, and Weekly Journal Page.

You should also make a list of your top 10 favorite foods.

And of course, be sure to eat together as a family at least five times a week and exercise together at least three times a week for 30 minutes.

Possible Journal Topics

In writing about the following topics, you may need only the few lines in your Weekly Journal Page. However, if these topics generate further thought, you may find it helpful to write more extensively. Emotional eating is the most common reason why younger people gain weight. This week in your journals, focus on the feelings surrounding eating. What are your feelings when you're eating? Do you sometimes find that you are eating because you're lonely or sad or angry? If you remember these feelings, this is what we are talking about when we use the phrase "emotional eating." The key to overcoming emotional eating is to find a way to express your feelings—take the opportunity in this week's journal to write down your feelings. You may find it difficult sometimes, but it's always better to let your feelings out than to keep them inside. If you need to, write down things in your journal that you could never tell anybody. Then try to think of three people who would understand if you did tell them. You're probably not the only person who feels this way. Write about the things that you're going through.

If you want, discuss in writing one of the following subjects (read them aloud so family members can choose which to write about).

1. Why is it better to eat what I need to be healthy, not what I *feel* I need to be happy?

2. Do I eat sometimes because I need to feel loved? How does that work when I eat too much? Does that make it easier or harder to feel loved?

3. Do I ever make fun of myself, thinking that if I don't, somebody else will? How does behaving this way make me feel?

4. How do my portion sizes compare to what's on the label?

5. What can I do that will make me feel proud of myself?

6. How can I do more of the things that make me feel good, like talking to friends or taking care of a pet?

WHAT PARENTS SHOULD KNOW

Improving your child's self-esteem should be one of your first priorities.

According to the American Psychology Review, *when 10- and 11-year-olds were asked to rank pictures of kids with physical handicaps according to desirability as a friend, they ranked obese kids lower than kids in wheelchairs or kids with amputated limbs.*

Parents may feel guilty, sad, and anxious for their overweight child, but they often express these feelings in ways that hurt their child's self-esteem. Some parents scold or belittle their children for overeating, which only adds to the child's sense of being a failure. Some parents try to restrict their child's food intake without discussing it with the child, sending a message that says, "You're no good and I don't trust you," and at a deeper level, the more frightening message, "I'm trying to starve you."

Kids must understand that they are loved unconditionally and should not feel judged. They should not feel like they're losing weight only to please you.

How can you help?

→ *In the half hour you spend exercising with your child, talk and listen.*

→ *Make sure your child knows that you trust him or her to make good decisions away from home.*

→ *When you obsess about food, you teach your children to obsess. Try to model healthy behavior for your children.*

→ *Look for professional help if needed (see list on pages 249–250).*

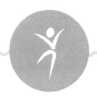

Chapter 7

WORKSHOP 3

Using Food Labels to Make Smart Decisions

The goal of this workshop is to learn how to make careful, intelligent decisions about the foods you eat. The good news is that all the information you need is at your fingertips, printed on food labels. You'll learn how to make a meal plan—and that the difference between a healthy diet and an unhealthy diet is knowing what to say yes to, what to say no to, and what to limit.

Start by totaling up the number of points everybody earned last week on your Weekly Point Charts. Then tally everyone's points on the Family Reward Chart. Ask the younger children how they feel about being rewarded for the good things they've done during the week—many younger kids are used to simply receiving things and aren't familiar with the idea of earning them. Older kids need praise as much as younger kids, and sometimes feel they don't get enough credit or recognition for the things they do. They also may not realize that when they skip an exercise session or binge on something unhealthy, they are only hurting themselves.

Do any family members have anything they want to bring to the table or share from their Weekly Journal Pages? Any questions about what you've learned so far? Comments, compliments, complaints?

Then read aloud from the following:

READ-ALOUD
FOOD FOR THOUGHT

Understand What You Are Eating (or Drinking)

Martin was five years old and too young to begin a regular exercise program. The son of a single working mother, he weighed nine pounds at birth. His mother, Melissa, breast-fed him until he was two years old. Melissa was average height and weight, as was Martin's father, Thomas, and yet Martin was as tall as a typical eight-year-old and weighed 72 pounds. Martin was much taller than would be expected based on his parents' heights, because overeating and becoming overweight had stimulated the secretion of hormones and growth factors. Melissa was concerned.

"He's always hungry, and thirsty, too" she explained to her doctor over the phone. "He drinks a lot, but it's just juice."

Martin's exam included a physical examination; forms to fill out regarding Martin's attitudes toward food, how much exercise he got, and how much television he watched; and "quality of life" questions to explore his mental health and the possibility of depression. More information surfaced during his interview. Martin watched several hours of television a day. Martin and his daily babysitter did little in the way of physical activity—the sitter watched over him as he played with his toys and sometimes watched television with him. He wasn't playing much with other kids, which can help a child be more active.

Martin and his mother met with a dietitian, and Martin began a new program. He was only allowed to watch an hour of television a day, with no eating during TV watching. More importantly, he was allowed only eight ounces of juice a day, and was given water to drink instead. The dietitian showed Melissa on the labels of the juices Martin had been drinking that most of them were sweetened with high-fructose corn syrup, a sugar the body digests very differently from other sugars and has been known to lead to weight gain. Some of the "juices" had as many as 160 to 170 calories in an eight-ounce serving. Even the 100 percent fruit juice contained 120 calories in an eight-ounce serving, and Martin was drinking up to 10 glasses a day—an astounding 1,200 calories and 260 grams of sugar just from juice. Melissa had made the same mistake a lot of parents make, assuming that giving Martin a glass of apple juice was good for him. But in terms of sugar intake, Martin was consuming the equivalent of 26 apples a day, without the fiber in apples, which, among other benefits, limits how fast sugar is absorbed.

Other changes were made. His sitter was asked to take him to the park instead of sitting around the house all day. Melissa enrolled him in a play group that gave him a chance to run around and chase after other kids. In the first three months of his new regimen, Martin didn't gain a pound, which, for a growing child, is the same as losing weight for an adult.

One of the simplest, yet most powerful changes we can make is being aware of the resources available to help us make wiser, more informed choices. One resource already in everybody's home is the label on the food we buy. Mindful eating means paying attention to information already at our fingertips. If Martin's mother had read the labels on the fruit juices he was drinking, she could have seen how many calories her son was getting from juice. It might have helped, however, if the label had mentioned that the 26 grams of sugar per serving he was getting equaled 6½ teaspoons of sugar.

It's easy to just see the large print on the front of the bottle that boasts of vitamin C or "real fruit juice" and not look at the tiny information label.

These days we need to know, more than ever, exactly what it is we're eating. Where nutrition is concerned, knowledge truly is power. Food labels can be confusing. What are niacin, thiamin, riboflavin, or folic acid, and what do they do? What are sodium, potassium, calcium, phosphorus, iodine, magnesium, iron, zinc, or copper, and why do we need to eat them?

The big words shouldn't intimidate us. These are all just vitamins and minerals we need as part of our diet (for a more detailed explanation of what they do, see pages 244–246). For losing weight, we need to pay attention primarily to three things on any food label—portion sizes, sugar content, and fat content.

Sugar is a carbohydrate. Carbohydrates, including sugars, starches, cellulose (or fiber), and other substances, are derived mainly from plants. Sugar comes from sugar cane, sugar beets, and corn, and occurs naturally in honey; different forms include sucrose, dextrose, turbinado, glucose, corn syrup, or high-fructose corn syrup.

While sugar is certainly tasty and can provide some fuel, too much damages teeth and it encourages us to fill up on sugary non-nutritious foods. It can also cause our blood sugar levels to "spike" and then drop quickly, leaving us hungrier afterward.

On a food label, the total carbohydrates are divided into sugars and fiber. Fiber (cellulose) comes from the cell walls of the plant cells we eat and can't be digested because it doesn't dissolve in water, passing instead through our system. It does important jobs, helping us regulate our bowel movements and protecting us from certain kinds of cancer. Fiber is good for you and does not lead to weight gain.

The carbohydrate to worry about is sugar, which we take in primarily in the form of sucrose or refined cane sugar, which then breaks down into glucose or blood sugar, the substance that supplies us with energy. In processed foods, the other source of sugar to be concerned about is listed among the ingredients on the label as "high-fructose corn syrup," or sometimes just "corn syrup."

Natural sugars in fruits are often combined with proteins, vitamins, or minerals, while refined sugars don't have these nutrients mixed in. This is why dietitians describe refined sugars as "empty" calories. The other danger of sugar is that we like the taste of it so much that we want to eat a lot of it. You may think that honey or fruit juice is healthier than white sugar, but the calorie count is the same—although unrefined sugars may be slightly better because sometimes other nutrients accompany them. Often food manufacturers put lots of sugar in foods that also have lots of fat, a dangerous double-whammy.

In small amounts, fat itself is not bad, and we need fat in our diets. According to the book *The Most Complete Food Counter*, fat supplies the fatty acids we need to manufacture hormones, cushions our organs, carries fat-soluble vitamins to different parts of the body, keeps us warm, and slows down digestion to make us feel full. And there *is* a difference between types of fat. Healthy fats from avocados, nuts, fish, and olive oil help remove cholesterol from our artery walls, improving blood flow. You will find unhealthy fats in hydrogenated vegetable oils, which are used in processed foods, and in milk, meat, and cheese. These fats can add cholesterol to our artery walls, restricting blood flow, which is why we limit these foods and choose low-fat milk.

We should get only about 30 percent of our daily calories from fat, and most of us greatly exceed that. Eating too much fat can cause heart disease, high blood pressure, or diabetes. One fat gram has nine calories, while a gram of carbohydrate or protein has only four calories—so you can see why everyone should be eating a limited amount of fat per day.

By looking at food labels, we can choose wisely between foods when we're shopping. If two foods appeal to us, but one is high in fat and sugar and the other is not, we can buy the one that's better for us—or if they both have too much fat and sugar, we can choose something else. Knowing how much fat there is in butter or cheese, we can use less of it when we make our sandwiches. If we're offered two choices for dessert, one high in refined sugars, like pie, and the other rich in natural sugars, like a piece of fruit, we can choose the dessert that's better for us, or have just a small bite of pie.

We don't need to analyze every food we eat every second of the day. We only need to keep an eye on fats, sugars, and portion sizes. With a little practice, we can all learn how to make a smart choice each time we eat or feel hungry.

Check-in

Everybody should discuss the previous week's workshop and briefly review what you learned. Family members should feel free to ask any questions, make suggestions, or air complaints. Anyone who wants to share something from his or her journal can do so. Then discuss in general terms:

1. What is fat?

2. Why does it taste so good?

3. Why is it at the top of the food pyramid?

4. What are the benefits of eating fat?

5. What are the consequences of eating too much fat?

6. Where do healthy fats come from?

7. Why are they healthy?

8. Where do unhealthy fats come from?

9. Why are they unhealthy?

10. Where is sugar?

11. Why is sugar bad for us?

12. Is there a difference between good and bad sugars?

Activity 1: Figuring Out Food Labels

For this activity, you will need clear plastic sandwich bags, measuring spoons, and a large container of vegetable shortening (such as Crisco).

Look at the typical food label (from a box of Cheerios) in Figure 7.1. Discuss the parts of the food label and the information they contain:

Serving size: the manufacturer's recommended portion. Be sure to compare serving sizes when food shopping. If two foods have the same number of calories per serving, but one serving size is larger than the other, the one with the larger serving size will have fewer calories per ounce.

Calories: how many calories in a serving.

Calories from fat: a good indicator of how healthy the food is—the closer this number is to the total calories in a serving, the fattier the food.

Percent daily values: how this food will fit into your daily diet plan. Remember that these are based on daily values recommended for adults. The reference values at the bottom tell you the government recommendations based on a 2,000- and a 2,500-calorie diet. Most kids need less than 2,000 calories. (See Table 7.2 on page 103.)

Total fat: on the first line of the percent daily value section. The amount of fat is shown in grams and as a percentage based on the Recommended Daily Allowance for adults.

Sugars: listed in the percent daily value section. The amount of sugar is shown in grams.

Vitamins: listed as a percentage based on the Recommended Daily Allowance for adults. In the label in Figure 7.1, one serving of this item will provide 25 percent of the vitamin C recommended for an adult for one day. Only two vitamins, A and C, and two minerals, calcium and iron, are required on a food label. Many labels list more nutrients.

Nutrition Facts

Serving Size 1 cup (30 g)
Servings Per Container About 10

Amount Per Serving

Calories 110   Calories from Fat 10

	% Daily Value*
Total Fat 1 g	**2%**
Saturated Fat 0 g	**0%**
Cholesterol	**0%**
Sodium	**10%**
Total Carbohydrate	**8%**
Dietary Fiber 3 g	**10%**
Sugars 6 g	
Protein 3 g	

Vitamin A 25% • Vitamin C 25%
Calcium 4% • Iron 45%

* Percent Daily Values are based on a 2,000 calorie diet. Your daily values might be higher or lower depending on your calorie needs:

	Calories:	2,000	2,500
Total Fat	Less than	65 g	80 g
Sat Fat	Less than	20 g	25 g
Cholesterol	Less than	300 mg	300 mg
Sodium	Less than	2,400 mg	2,400 mg
Total Carbohydrate		300 g	375 g
Dietary Fiber		25 g	30 g

Calories per gram:
Fat 9 • Carbohydrate 4 • Protein 4

FIGURE 7.1

Talk about the meaning of some common terms seen on food packaging:

Calorie free: less than 5 calories per serving.

Low calorie: 40 calories or less per serving.

Fat free: less than half a gram per serving.

Reduced fat, less fat: at least 25 percent less fat than the higher-fat version.

Low fat: 3 grams or less per serving.

Lean: less than 19 grams total fat, less than 4 grams saturated fat, and less than 95 mg cholesterol (refers to seafood, meat, or poultry).

Extra lean: less than 5 grams total fat, less than 2 grams saturated fat, and less than 95 mg cholesterol (refers to seafood, meat, or poultry).

Cholesterol free: less than 20 milligrams of cholesterol and 2 grams or less of fat.

Light: one-third fewer calories and 50 percent less fat than a similar product.

High fiber: 5 grams or more of fiber per serving.

Good source of fiber: 2.5 to 4.9 grams of fiber per serving.

Sugar free: less than 0.5 grams of sugar per serving.

Good source of: 10 to 19 percent of the Daily Value (based on a 2,000-calorie diet) per serving.

Low sodium: 140 milligrams or less per serving.

On the food label, sugar and fat are measured in grams. But what do these amounts of sugar or fat actually look like?

Let's compare a candy bar and a granola bar. A chocolate bar with almonds (1½-ounce size) has 18 grams of sugar, and a granola bar has 6 grams of sugar. One teaspoon of sugar is equal to 4 grams. This means that the candy bar has 4½ teaspoons of sugar, and the granola bar has 1½ teaspoons of sugar. For both the candy bar and the granola bar, use measuring teaspoons to measure the amount of sugar into separate bags. Compare the bags. Which has more sugar? How much more?

Now let's look at the amount of fat in the same candy bar and granola bar. (On a food label, be sure to check serving size—sometimes a serving is only half a candy bar!) The candy bar has 14 grams of fat, and the granola bar has 3 grams of fat. One teaspoon of fat is equal to 4 grams. So the candy bar has 3½ teaspoons of fat, and the granola bar has ¾ teaspoon of fat. With a measuring teaspoon, measure these amounts of shortening into two separate clear plastic bags. Compare the bags for the candy bar and the granola bar. Which of the two do you think is healthier to eat? How does it make you feel when you think about eating the amount of fat in the candy bar?

If you were shopping for granola bars or other snack foods, how would you choose between healthy and unhealthy versions?

Now examine the amounts of sugar and fat in some other common foods by doing the following exercises.

PART 1. See how much sugar is in the drinks in the following list, which you may have in your cupboard or refrigerator. For each drink, measure the number of teaspoons of sugar into separate clear plastic bags.

	Grams of sugar	Teaspoons of sugar
Soda (12-oz. can)	40 g	10.0 tsp.
Fruit juice (12-oz. can)	37 g	9.5 tsp.
Unsweetened iced tea (12-oz. glass)	0	0

Now measure out the amount of sugar in a 64-ounce Big Gulp soda, which has 213 grams, or 53 teaspoons, of sugar. You may need a bowl! That's a lot of sugar, isn't it?

PART 2. Let's do the same for some popular high-fat foods. In the following list, measure out the number of teaspoons of fat for each food into separate plastic bags.

	Grams of fat	Teaspoons of fat
Ice cream (½ c.)	10 g	2.5 tsp.
Crackers (15 crackers)	20 g	5.0 tsp.
Pepperoni pizza (1 slice)	14 g	3.5 tsp.

PART 3. See how much sugar you would consume in a day if you ate all of the following. Measure it out. Again, you may need a bowl!

	Grams of sugar	Teaspoons of sugar
Syrup (¼ c.) with your pancakes	53 g	13 tsp.
3 sodas (12 oz. each)	120 g	30 tsp.
10 cookies	40 g	10 tsp.
1 fruit yogurt (8 oz.)	40 g	10 tsp.
1 glass of juice (8 oz.)	25 g	6 tsp.
2 candy bars (1½ oz. each)	36 g	9 tsp.
1 slice of cake	47 g	12 tsp.
1 scoop of ice cream (½ c.)	16 g	4 tsp.
TOTAL	377 g	94 tsp.

Finally, measure 34 teaspoons (136 grams) of sugar into a plastic bag. This is the amount most teenagers eat in a day. Now measure 10 teaspoons (40 grams) into another plastic bag. This is the amount of sugar an average teenager should be eating in a day.

Then measure out 30 grams of fat, which is 7½ teaspoons. This is the amount of fat an adult should have in a day. Many kids and adults eat twice as much or more. Add another 30 grams of shortening to the bag and let kids squish it around in their fingers. Pick up the bag containing 34 teaspoons of sugar and hold it and the 60 grams of fat side by side. Do you really want to eat this much sugar and fat every day?

You can lower the fat in your diet if you follow these tips:

→ Add herbs and spices to food to intensify the flavor.

→ Replace butter with low-fat margarine.

→ Eat chicken and fish more often than you eat red meat.

→ Eat at least one fruit or vegetable every meal. (Remember that in our food guide pyramid, starchy foods such as potatoes, peas, and corn do *not* count as vegetables.)

→ Bake, broil, or steam food rather than fry.

→ Try sorbet or sherbet instead of ice cream.

→ Enjoy nonfat flavored yogurt.

→ Choose nonfat salad dressing.

→ Rinse cooked meat in running water before adding it to a recipe in order to remove some of the excess fat that emerges while cooking.

→ Buy natural peanut butter and pour off half the oil before stirring.

→ Blot up the excess oil from a slice of pizza with a paper towel before you eat it.

→ Choose skim or 1 percent milk.

What about Sugar and Fat Substitutes?

Is your child a soda guzzler? You're right to be concerned. Three sodas a day add up to more than 120 grams of sugar—which can lead to a clear and measurable increased risk of obesity, high blood pressure, high cholesterol, and type 2 diabetes, if maintained over time. Think about it this way: The child who drinks three sodas a day for 10 years will have consumed nearly *half a ton* of sugar.

So you may be tempted to steer your child toward drinks that are artificially sweetened, such as diet sodas, Crystal Lite, or Wyler's Light. But using an artificial sweetener to lower calorie intake may be a case of trading one risk for another. The threat of developing cancer from beverages containing artificial sweeteners is considerably more remote than the threat of obesity-related problems—but it remains a trade-off.

Sugar substitutes were invented primarily to help people with diabetes. Although eating foods with sugar substitutes will not contribute to the overall calories a person consumes, some experts believe that eating too many of these products may be harmful. Often there will be a continued craving for the sweet foods if a sugar substitute is given. It is also common for children to consume diet drinks instead of milk, which results in insufficient calcium consumption and can potentially lead to osteoporosis. The recommended maximum amount of sugar substitutes is 1 to 2 servings of foods sweetened with these per day.

Here are the different types of artificial sweeteners.

Saccharin. In the 1970s the Food and Drug Administration attempted to ban this sweetener (discovered in 1879 at Johns Hopkins University) after studies found increased rates of bladder cancer in laboratory rats. Manufacturers maintained that consumers would have to consume huge amounts of saccharin to match the amounts ingested by the rats in the studies. Congress now requires only warning labels.

Aspartame. The most popular artificial sweetener, discovered in 1969 in Germany, is marketed as Equal or Nutra-Sweet and is made from artichokes. Among the more than 600 studies of aspartame, one test linked aspartame to slightly increased rates of brain tumors in rats. Side effects may include headaches or dizziness.

Sorbitol. You may find this modified sugar molecule in confections—it gives foods a sweet taste but cannot be absorbed by the gastrointestinal tract. A French chemist discovered it in 1872 in berries of a mountain ash tree. The primary side effect is diarrhea, when taken in excessive amounts.

Sucralose. This sweetener, discovered in 1976 by British researchers, is sold as Splenda. It's produced by chlorinating sugar, tastes like sugar, and is stable enough to be used in baking. Too few human studies have been conducted to access the risks, but in rats, mice, and rabbits, sucralose may cause shrunken thymus glands and other problems. A Food and Drug Administration document says that sucralose has a weak potential to cause cancer in animals, while results of other studies are inconclusive. At present, dietitians recommend Sucralose more often than the other sweeteners. However, too few studies have been conducted for us to know the ultimate risks.

How about fat? Yes, an artificial fat exists—made from plastic. This indigestible fat substitute, called Olestra, has brought about 20,000 complaints to the Food and Drug Administration, more than all other food additives in history combined, and many manufacturers are pulling it from shelves as the result of poor sales. Side effects may include diarrhea, incontinence, cramping, bleeding, and an oily "leakage." Avoid foods with olestra—check labels carefully.

Rather than encouraging your family to eat foods with questionable ingredients, you should offer them a diet with proper portions of whole grains, fresh fruits, vegetables, meat, fish, and dairy products. Discourage your child's sweet tooth, or teach your child to satiate it with natural sugars such as those found in fresh fruits. The beverages of choice for children are milk and water, with one serving of fruit juice per day.

Activity 2: Making a Personal Pyramid

In the previous workshop you familiarized yourselves with the various portion sizes and practiced measuring out portions in your favorite bowls and dishes. The food guide pyramid also showed you the proper ratios and explained servings in a general way. Now it's time to get more specific. You need a variety of foods every day. You don't want to skip meals, which slows down your metabolism because your body thinks it's being starved. Each meal should be part of a larger menu plan. You need to know how many servings of each food group you need each day, then maintain a healthy balanced diet. The number of servings you need will vary according to age, gender, and activity level.

In your Weekly Food Log you kept track of all the food you ate. Look at the food you ate yesterday, and use the following list to calculate the number of servings you consumed from each food group.

SINGLE SERVING SIZES ACCORDING TO FOOD GROUP

Bread, Cereal, Rice, Pasta, and Starchy Vegetable Group

    1 slice of bread

    ½ bagel, English muffin, hamburger/hot dog bun

    6-inch pita bread

    ¾ cup unsweetened dry cereal or ½ cup sugar frosted cereal

    ½ cup cooked cereal, rice, or pasta

    5 or 6 small crackers, low-fat or nonfat

    ½ cup corn, peas, mashed potatoes, yams/sweet potatoes (plain)

    1 cup winter squash

    1 small baked or broiled potato

    3 cups popcorn (popped, no fat added or low-fat microwave)

    1 corn tortilla, 6 inches

    1 flour tortilla, 7 to 8 inches

    1 waffle, 4½ inches square, reduced fat

Vegetables

    1 cup raw vegetables

    ½ cup cooked vegetables

½ cup vegetable juice

½ cup tomato sauce

Fruit

1 small fresh fruit

½ cup fruit juice

¼ cup dried fruit

1 frozen 100% fruit juice bar

½ cup fruit, canned, in water, in juice or extra-light syrup

Milk and Yogurt

1 cup skim, ½% fat, or 1% fat milk, or nonfat or low-fat buttermilk

⅓ cup nonfat dry milk or ½ cup evaporated skim milk

1 cup nonfat or low-fat flavored yogurt or plain yogurt

Lean Protein (1 ounce protein)

1 ounce lean poultry, beef, pork, lamb, game, all shellfish, and fish with no skin and/or all excess fat cut off.

1 ounce low-fat or nonfat deli meats (3 grams fat or less per ounce)

1 ounce low-fat or nonfat cheese (3 grams fat or less per ounce)

½ cup cooked dried beans, lentils, or other legumes

2 egg whites

¼ cup nonfat or low-fat cottage cheese

1 lean turkey hot dog (3 grams fat or less per ounce)

Medium-Fat Protein (1 ounce protein + 1 fat serving, which is equal to 5 grams fat)

1 cup soy milk

1 ounce fried chicken

1 ounce feta or mozzarella cheese

¼ cup ricotta cheese

High-Fat Protein (1 ounce protein + 2 fat servings, which is equal to 10 grams fat)

1 ounce cheese

1 ounce processed sandwich meats, such as bologna or salami

2 tablespoons natural peanut butter

10 peanuts or 6 mixed nuts, almonds, cashews or 4 pecan or walnut halves

1 regular hot dog (beef or pork)

Fats and Sweets (1 serving equals 45 calories, which is equal to 10 grams sugar or 5 grams fat)

1 teaspoon regular or 1 tablespoon reduced-fat oil, margarine, butter, or mayonnaise

1 tablespoon salad dressing or 2 tablespoons reduced-fat salad dressing

1 tablespoon cream cheese or 2 tablespoons reduced-fat cream cheese

⅛ avocado

½ cup light or reduced-fat ice cream or ¼ cup ice cream

2 teaspoons tahini paste

1 teaspoon lard or shortening

2 tablespoons chitterlings, boiled

2 small cookies

½ frosted cupcake

½ sweet roll or pan dulce (Mexican sweet bread)

Note that foods such as French fries, onion rings, potato chips, candy bars, chewing gum, fruit leather, frozen ice pops (those that are not 100 percent fruit), and Coke and other sodas, are not included on this list. The list consists only of foods that are *recommended*. If you're wondering how many servings of these types of foods you're allowed—ideally, none.

Fats and sweets should be used sparingly because other foods already contain so much fat and sugar. For instance, 10 French fries count as one serving from the grain group plus one serving from the fat group. One hot dog counts as one protein serving and one fat serving. One serving of ice cream counts as one dairy serving plus one or two fat servings, depending on the fat content.

When you've finished calculating the number of servings you ate, it's time to sort them into food groups. Draw a blank food pyramid (or use a copy of the one on page 232) and make one mark for every serving you ate in the appropriate box in the pyramid. If you don't know where a certain food you ate belongs, talk it over with your family and make your best guess. For example, if you ate cereal with milk and a banana for breakfast, for cereal make a mark in the grain group at the base of the pyramid, for milk make a mark in the dairy group, and for banana make a mark in the fruit group. Often people who think they're eating healthily are surprised to see that their diet is far from ideal.

Be sure to pay attention to what kinds of foods you're eating within the larger classifications. Low-fat or nonfat milk is better than whole milk. Unsweetened cereal is better than sweetened cereal. Whole grains are better than refined grains. Lean protein is better than high-fat protein; for example, if you consume a high-fat protein, you are also consuming 2 fat servings (see page 100) for every ounce of protein that you eat, and these servings of fat need to be counted toward your daily total of fat. As everyone builds a personal food pyramid, a picture of each individual's diet begins to emerge.

Compare the pyramid you filled in with the recommended number of servings in the food guide pyramid. (Obviously, you can't compare fat/sweet servings to the food pyramid, because it just says "eat sparingly.")

1. In which areas did you eat more than the recommended number of servings?

2. In which areas did you eat less than the recommended number of servings?

3. What do you think it means if your diet has varied from the recommended ratios?

4. Can you think of two ways you could eat better?

Next, add up the number of servings you ate for the other six days of the week, and then add together all seven days' worth of servings to arrive at a weekly total for each food group. Divide that weekly total by seven to arrive at your daily average. How do those numbers compare to the food guide pyramid?

The food guide pyramid is only a general guide. You'll want to fine-tune what you eat to your own body. Table 7.2 will tell you the number of servings you should be eating for your personal age and gender group. The table makes

SAMPLE DIETS FOR A DAY

	Overweight children, ages 5–8	Overweight children, ages 9–11	Adult women & older adults above age 70	Overweight children, ages 12–14	Adult men	Teen girls & athletic women	Teen boys & athletic men
Calorie level	About 1,200	About 1,500	About 1,600	About 1,800	About 2,000	About 2,200	About 2,800
Grain group servings	4	5	6	8	9	9	11
Vegetable group servings	3	3	3	3	4	4	5
Fruit group servings	2	2	2	4	4	3	4
Milk group servings	2	2	2 to 3	3	3	2 to 3	2 to 3
Protein group servings	4 oz.	4 oz.	5 oz.	6 oz.	6 oz.	6 oz.	7 oz.
Total fat allowed	40 g	46 g	53 g	60 g	67 g	73 g	93 g

TABLE 7.2

allowances for adults who are "athletic," which is defined as engaging in at least five hours per week of moderate to vigorous physical activity.

Although we are focusing on the number of servings, Table 7.2 also includes some other useful information. It shows the calorie levels, as well as the total fat allowed, for each age, gender, and (for adults) activity level. These calorie levels are based on your choosing low-fat, lean foods from the five major food groups and using fats, oils, and sweets sparingly. For example, if you are an 11-year-old boy, you are allowed 1,500 calories and 46 grams of fat. Some of this fat will come from the foods you are eating from the five main groups. So to meet your allowance of 46 grams of fat per day, you must eat sparingly of high-fat foods and foods in the fats, oils, and sweets category.

Let's return to the daily average of servings for each food group that you calculated based on your Weekly Food Log. Compare those numbers of servings with the recommended number for your age, gender, and (for adults) activity level in Table 7.2. For fat servings, one serving equals 5 grams of fat. So to compare your average daily fat servings to the allowance in Table 7.2, multiply your number of fat servings by 5. Now ask again—how does your typical day's diet differ from what's recommended for your age and gender? What do you need to change to make your diet more closely resemble the recommended diet?

Note that you should start by eating the number of servings recommended for your age, gender, and (for adults) activity level. If you find that you are either not losing weight, or losing weight too quickly (more than two pounds per week), then adjust your number of servings accordingly.

Activity 3: Your Personal Meal Plan

Using My Daily Food Guide Pyramid from page 233 (a copy should be in everyone's folder), create your own personal meal plan. Look at Table 7.2 to see how many servings of each food group you need, and write down the numbers of servings in the corresponding boxes in the pyramid. In the box for fats/sweets, write down the number of fat grams shown in the "total fat allowed" row of Table 7.2.

The next step involves the food cards on pages 234–239, which the leader should have prepared before the meeting. The leader needs to make enough copies of each food group card for each team member. It is a good idea to use a different color paper for each food group. (If you have access to a color printer, you can print out the cards in color from www.kidshape.com.) Since there are four copies of each card on a sheet of paper, for a team of two adults and two children, the leader should make the following number of copies:

Food group	Sheet color	Number of copies
Grains	Yellow	8
Vegetables	Green	4
Fruit	Orange	3
Milk, Yogurt	Blue	3
Protein	Red	3
Fats, Sweets	Pink	6

These numbers can be adjusted based on the number of participants. Once the cards have been copied, cut the sheets apart.

Deal yourself one card for every serving from each food group, as shown in My Daily Food Guide Pyramid, which you just created. For the purpose of this activity, deal yourself one fats/sweets card for every 10 grams of fat shown in the fats/sweets box in your pyramid. In other words, divide the fat grams by 10, rounding to the closet whole number. For example, a 12-year-old child is allowed 60 grams of fat and gets 6 fats/sweets cards.

The important thing is that everyone has an individual set of cards that fits that person's specific meal plan. If your personal meal plan allows for five grain servings a day, give yourself five grain cards. If you're allowed four protein servings, give yourself four protein cards, and so on.

Once everybody has a set of cards, together draw up a menu for a typical day by writing down everything you might have for all three meals, including snacks. Using the Family Meal Plan worksheet from page 240 (the leader should have this form in his or her folder), write down a sample menu for an entire day. For each meal and snack, place a check in the correct food group box. Most meals will have more than one box checked. For example, a breakfast of ½ cup of Cheerios, with 1 cup of low-fat milk and ½ banana, will yield one check mark in the grains group, one in the fruit group, and one in the milk/yogurt group (see sample checks on the Family Meal Plan worksheet). Once you complete your menu, count up each of your check marks for each food group. The check marks in each food group should equal the number of servings listed on your meal plan and the number of cards for your daily allowance. For example, your menu should have three milk/yogurt checks if your meal plan has three milk/yogurt servings listed. Obviously, an adult may have more cards from each food group than a child to spread over the day. The best way to use the Family Meal Plan is to plan the same basic meal for the whole family, but to allow more servings, from the grain group for example, at that meal for the adult than for the child.

Once you've got your menu planned, read the ingredients out loud, starting with breakfast, and for each item on the menu, lay down the corresponding food card in a row on the table in front of you. You might even want to write down on the card what food item and portion size that card represents. If you've planned your menu perfectly, all family members should have laid down all their cards by the end of the day's menu, without any gaps in any of their rows. When you're finished, discuss the following questions:

1. If you have leftover cards, what are they?

2. If you ran out of cards in one group, which group was that?

3. Based on your leftover cards, what foods do you need to add to your menu?

4. Based on the cards you ran out of, what foods do you need to subtract from your menu?

5. How can you more evenly distribute your food groups across all three meals?

Now is the time to review your homework assignment from your last workshop, the list you made of your 10 favorite foods. For each item on your list, find the corresponding food card. Discuss the following questions:

1. Can you create healthy meals from the kinds of foods you like to eat?

2. How could you work your favorite foods into healthy meals?

3. How do you feel when you eat your favorite foods?

4. Are they high in fat?

5. Are they high in sugar?

6. Can you think of ways to substitute lower-fat or lower-sugar versions of your favorite foods?

One of last week's goals was to measure food portions. What did you learn when you measured your portions during the week? How accurate were you? Are your portion sizes bigger or smaller than you expected? What surprised you?

Weekly Goals

On your Weekly Goals form, fill in the following goals:

1. I will include a new vegetable (_____) in a meal.

2. I will eat a low-fat food item.

3. I will do a physically active chore around the house.

4. I will have a turn-off-the-TV day.

Homework Assignment

Keep track of everything you eat and drink during the week by filling in your Weekly Food Log. Be sure to keep up with your Weekly Activity Log, Weekly Journal Page, and Weekly Goals.

Now that you know how to read food labels, go through your cabinets and refrigerator as a family to find healthy and non-healthy, high-sugar, high-fat foods in your house. Throw away open packages and take any unopened packages to your local food bank, if you wish. Then take a trip to the grocery store to replace the discarded food items with healthier choices. Kids should go grocery shopping with the adults and help choose low-fat, low sugar foods for the whole family from the supermarket shelves. Remember to read the food labels!

As usual, you should eat together as a family at least five times a week and exercise together at least three times a week for 30 minutes.

Possible Journal Topics

Read aloud the following questions, so family members can choose which topics they want to discuss in their journals.

1. What is the smallest change I can make to be healthier?

2. What changes are easy to make? Why are they easy? What changes are more difficult? Why?

3. What makes my favorite foods my favorites, and what are the alternatives?

4. What does a cup of cereal look like in our bowls?

5. What is a serving size of orange juice, and what does it look like in our glasses?

6. How can I know what foods to say yes to?

7. How should I say no to the foods that aren't good for me?

WHAT PARENTS SHOULD KNOW

It's up to parents to set limits on a child's eating, but that's easier said than done. You've probably already tried and met with some resistance. As children grow, so does their desire for independence and autonomy. But being overweight is a sign that your children are having trouble setting limits for themselves. Here are some simple ways to set limits.

Television. Limit the amount of television they can watch—one hour a day is the recommended maximum.

Types of foods. Limit the types of foods you have in the house, particularly snacks children can help themselves to. Replace snacks high in fat or sugar with healthy ones such as fresh fruit, sliced vegetables, or graham crackers. Kids need to feel in control of their own bodies. They can choose from the healthy snacks what they want to eat and feel responsible for the weight they lose.

Time in restaurants. Limit the amount of time you eat in restaurants. This will mean cooking more meals at home, where you can control the content and the portion sizes of the foods you eat. If you do eat in restaurants, find ones where healthy choices can be made.

Teasing. Ask siblings not to tease their overweight brother or sister, and ask overweight kids not to make comments at their own expense. Having a sense of humor is good, but self-deprecation reinforces a child's negative self-image. Overweight kids should be treated just like any other member of the family, which includes eating the same foods. Don't single out overweight children by giving them different foods from the rest of the family.

Your own negativity. Don't punish a child for something he or she ate, because it will only make her want to eat more. Praise your children when they measure their foods or write in their journals. Accept and honor your child, without believing that your child being overweight is a reflection on your parenting skills. If you act ashamed or embarrassed, your child will know and be strongly affected.

Alone time. Spend time with your children, and take them for walks or swims if you have an unscheduled afternoon.

Silence. Don't let things go unsaid. Ask your kids how they feel and wait for the answer. Encourage them to express their feelings. Set an example by talking about your own feelings and expressing your own doubts, fears, or misgivings. If your child has a hard time talking to you, consider bringing him to a therapist where he'll feel free to talk. If you feel like a failure as a parent, or if your child's weight problem seems like an issue you cannot handle or face, you may wish to speak to a therapist yourself.

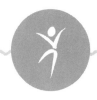

CHAPTER 8

WORKSHOP 4

Move It to Lose It

This workshop will help you learn about the importance of regular physical activities, and your own body image. We will focus on developing an enjoyable fitness routine, which will include activities that you can do by yourself as well as those that you can do together as a team. You'll also learn about how to monitor your heart rate and choose healthy snacks, and the importance of drinking plenty of water.

To begin, all family members should total up the points they earned since the last workshop on their Weekly Point Charts. Then tally and record everyone's points on the Family Reward Chart. Praise everyone for earning points and for trying hard.

Then share how you're feeling about the program so far. What does each person like the most about it? The least? Is there anything you want to repeat that might still be confusing you? Is there anything you think hasn't gotten enough attention, or too much? Does anyone have anything they want to share from their Weekly Journal Pages? Does anyone have a related topic they want to bring up or discuss?

Then read aloud from the following:

Time to Get Moving!

Graham worked in the film industry, and his wife, Rachel, stayed home with their daughter, Julia, 11. One day Rachel brought Julia in to see her doctor, concerned because Julia had gained 30 pounds. Julia claimed she wasn't getting teased about her weight at school, but seemed terribly self-conscious about her weight. Rachel was worried.

"I don't want to make Julia more self-conscious than she already is," Rachel said, "but I was just wondering how I can help her without constantly reminding her of the problem."

Rachel added that, although her own weight was normal, she had fought a weight problem her whole life. She didn't want Julia to suffer the way she had.

"I'm afraid I might have passed on my bad genes to my daughter," she said. "I've tried to keep Julia on a variety of diets. We even tried the Atkins diet, but nothing seems to work."

Rachel was told that the Atkins diet was not recommended for growing children and in fact posed some risks for them. The doctor then recommended a glucose challenge test that measured blood insulin and glucose levels. The tests revealed that Julia was suffering from hyperinsulinemia or excessively high blood insulin levels, associated with insulin resistance and a higher risk of type 2 diabetes.

This was why it was difficult for Julia to lose weight. In hyperinsulinemia, your body produces more insulin than it can use (it's caused by eating too much and too often for a long time without getting enough exercise). With high insulin levels, you feel hungrier than normal: Your body keeps saying, "Feed me, I'm starving," even when your stomach is full. Having too much insulin also prevents fat from breaking down and inhibits calorie-burning.

The doctor recommended that Julia restrict fats and processed carbohydrates and adopt a program of moderate exercise to get her weight and her hyperinsulinemia under control.

Julia immediately changed her diet and reduced the amount of television she watched each night from three hours to one. She joined a soccer team at school and began exercising regularly with her parents. As a result, she lost 15 pounds in four months, a perfect weight to maintain considering that she was growing.

Twenty-eight percent of U.S. adults do *no* physical activity during the day and another 42 percent get less than the recommended 30 minutes a day, according to the U.S. Department of Health and Human Services. This means a full 70 percent of us lead basically sedentary lives. And children in the United States spend as much time during a year watching television as they do attending school, reports a study in the *Archives of Pediatrics and Adolescent Medicine.*

Sedentary living (living without exercise) can lead to a group of serious illnesses and diseases that is sometimes called insulin resistance syndrome. A lack of exercise can contribute to heart problems, high blood fat and cholesterol, certain cancers, strokes, type 2 diabetes, and even depression. Insulin resistance syndrome accounts for more than half of doctor visits, ER visits, and prescription drug use, according to an article in *Endocrine Practice.*

The good news is that we can easily increase our activity: simply by opening our front door and going for a walk, or dancing to the radio indoors. There are countless ways to become active, and most of them are fun.

The problem is that we've invented so many ways to be inactive that are also fun, such as television, computers, and talking on the phone. Sometimes we feel we need to be inactive and relax because our days are so busy.

We might want to take our cue from nature—survival of the fittest is still the rule. A lion lazing on a rock in the sun will use his stored energy when he has to hunt. But the lion who gets fat, spending too much time lying in the sun gazing at the herds below, will sooner or later become too slow to catch his dinner. In nature, most animals have arrived at a balance between conserving energy and expending it to stay fit and healthy. But many people's lives are out of balance. The most energy we expend gathering our food supplies today is usually lifting the grocery bags from the shopping cart to the car.

The best way to lose weight and keep it off forever is through a combination of diet and exercise. We can increase activities that burn calories and decrease activities such as TV watching that allow calories to be stored as fat, while at the same time decreasing the calories we take in. We can lose weight simply by cutting calories or increasing our activity levels, but both together work much better and faster. The more we exercise, the more we can eat, and the more we cut back on calories, the less we need to exercise. The more we do both, the faster we'll lose weight.

Today most of us are rushing around to get everything done, and we all wish we had more time. In a way, time is money, but time is love too. Time is family and serenity.

Most health and fitness experts say that health risks decrease with 30 minutes of exercise daily. This is why we have all committed to a minimum of 30 minutes, three times a week (though more is good too).

Exercise will give us more energy and improve our moods. Long-term benefits sometimes feel invisible to us, but we know they're there: We will be greatly reducing the risks of serious diseases such as diabetes and heart disease. We will soon see weight loss. (And other good things will happen that we won't see: more HDL or good cholesterol in our blood, lower cholesterol, stronger bones.)

Exercise can be fun! It's not a punishment. It's a good thing we do for ourselves. It can be tough to get started, which is why exercising with a support group is so important. It is much easier to motivate ourselves if we have somebody exercising with us, or if we've promised somebody we'll join them. It's also easier when we know we're not doing it only for our own benefit, but also because someone we love and care about needs our help. It's more fun when we know we'll have support and encouragement and someone to talk to along the way. Families are ideally suited to exercising together.

Everyone may have a different idea of what to do, and we can take turns choosing. Exercise doesn't just mean things like push-ups and pull-ups. It includes hiking in the woods, walking a dog, bicycling, roller skating, jumping rope, or dancing—whatever gets our hearts pumping.

The goal is to establish a lifestyle change that can benefit us all for the rest of our lives. We can develop new skills or learn new games to play. Parents can change lazy habits. Individually, we have only one goal, which is to do our best, every time we try. Our aim is to get better each week. We might measure our progress by how many push-ups, pull-ups, or sit-ups we can do, but a more important measure is how many days we keep working out and staying active. Eventually, we can stop counting—because we will have made daily activity a habit.

STOP

Check-in

Discuss what you like or dislike about physical activity, which activities are your favorites and which your least favorite. Talk about your best and worst moments physically, in sports or in gym class. Talk about your favorite professional athletes, if you have any, and the things they do to stay fit. Talk about all the forms of inactivity (TV, video games), what's appealing about them, and what's harmful. Discuss the following questions:

1. Why is watching so much television harmful? (Answer: It reduces time to be active; it lowers metabolism; it advertises fattening foods, particularly during children's programming.)

2. What is a calorie? (Answer: It's not a measure of fat, but rather a measure of heat, reflecting the amount of energy available from a given food when it's burned, just like a log in the fireplace. When you eat, your body stores the fuel it doesn't immediately need for later use—the fat you see when you look in the mirror is just stored fuel. The only way to get rid of stored fuel is to burn it through activity.)

3. How much fuel do we have to burn to lose weight? (Answer: Burning as few as 200 extra calories a day can be enough to start weight loss.)

4. What other benefits does exercise have, besides weight loss? (Answer: Exercise has a huge beneficial effect on our emotions and mental state. It also builds muscle at the same time that it burns fat.)

5. Why does exercise hurt sometimes? (Answer: The only way to build muscles is to overload them by giving them more work than they're used to. That means you have to do a little extra, jump higher, run farther or longer, pushing yourself just slightly beyond the comfort zone. Sometimes lactic acids build up in muscle tissues that have been overloaded, causing soreness, although massage and stretching can relieve that. When you overload your muscles, your body responds by growing more muscle cells to help carry the extra load. Remember that people often feel reluctant to exercise, but few people exercise and then regret having done it.)

Keeping Fit by Helping Out

The scope of health-promoting activities need not be restricted to more traditional exercises such as running, cycling, or swimming. While you still want to make time for aerobic exercise three times a week for 30 minutes, there are also benefits to be gained from simply including your child in your daily household chores, according to a report in the journal *Circulation*. Think of all the things you have to do each night before you can finally go to sleep. If you work outside the home, you are probably exhausted by the end of the day. Yet it may also be true that your children feel ignored while you plow through the cleaning and the laundry while picking up all the junk that gets strewn about the house on a routine day. By asking your children to help with the chores, you give them an opportunity to be more active. At the same time, working side-by-side with a parent allows them to gain self-confidence and self-esteem as they see the concrete contributions that they are making to the family.

What kinds of chores qualify will depend on how old your children are and where you live. If you own a home in a climate where it snows, you and your child can shovel the walk or the driveway. If you live in a city apartment, you may ask your child to take out the trash or sweep the floor. In many communities, washing the family car is a weekend ritual that provides both a great deal of physical activity and a visible end product your child can be proud of. In the end, children love to imitate the grown-ups they admire. Working together gives you an opportunity to be with your child and gives all of you more free time to spend on recreational activities. Additionally, you'll be teaching your child by example how to set goals, accomplish tasks, and earn the reward of a job well done.

Activity 1: Finding Your Heart Rate

There are two ways to know if you're exercising hard enough.

The first is to measure your heart rate. Practice by taking your resting heart rate. Take your first two fingers (not your thumb) of your right hand and place your fingertips at the corner of your right eye, then slide your fingers down until you reach the top of your neck and press in lightly. The throbbing you feel is your pulse. Count the number of times your heart beats while someone else counts off six seconds. Then multiply that number by 10—that's the number of times your heart is beating in a minute.

Write that number down.

Your target heart rate is a "moderately intense" level, between 50 and 70 percent of your maximum heart rate. To figure out your recommended maximum, subtract your age from 220. If you're 10, your maximum heart rate is 210 beats per minute. If you're 50, your maximum recommended heart rate is 170.

Divide the number you come up with by 2 to calculate 50 percent. Multiply it by 0.70 to determine what 70 percent is. Your goal when you exercise is to keep your heart rate between these two numbers for 30 minutes.

"KidShape has helped us understand the correlation between our eating habits and our self-esteem."

—KidShape parent

Now everybody walk up and down a flight of stairs as fast as you can for one minute. If you don't have a staircase, you can step on and off the front step, or do jumping jacks for one minute, whatever it takes to get you winded and out of breath. When one minute is up, immediately take your pulse again. Write that number down. Did you reach your targeted heart rate?

The other way to know if you're exercising hard enough is to try to carry on a conversation while you're working out. If you're so out of breath that you can't talk, you're working too hard, but if you're breathing so easily that you can sing, you're not working hard enough. Again, to get the maximum benefit, you will want to sustain this rate for at least 30 minutes.

Remember that the harder you work, the more calories you burn, as shown in Table 8.1.

CALORIES BURNED IN EXERCISE

Exercise (30 min.)	Calories you burn
Running at 5 mph	310
Running at 10 mph	500
Jumping rope for 30 minutes	420
Biking at 6 mph	120
Biking at 10 mph	180
Swimming medium	150
Swimming fast	360
Walking at 2 mph	90
Walking at 5 mph	210

TABLE 8.1

Activity 2: The Importance of Water

If walking up and down the stairs for a minute made you thirsty, pause for a glass of water. As you drink, take a moment to appreciate the importance of water. Every living thing needs water. When scientists look for evidence of life on other planets, they first look for water. Every chemical reaction that goes on inside your body requires water. Water is also how your body gets rid of the toxins that build up in your cells. When you feel thirsty, your body is telling you you're dehydrated. You should drink water with all your meals and snacks.

You want to work out hard enough to work up a sweat. Burning stored energy reserves during exercise will make your body temperature go up. You should drink water before, during, and after exercise to help your body recover and cool down. You should also get in the habit of drinking enough: As a general rule, active adults (16 years and older) should drink 64 ounces of water a day; active children (6 years and older) should drink 48 ounces.

Use your measuring cups and measure out the amount of water you need in a day. Try dividing the amount you need in a day into six glasses—that would be one glass with each meal, one with each snack, and one before bed. Often people mistake thirst for hunger. Drinking enough water helps you lose weight because it fills you up and suppresses this false hunger.

You will also want to drink additional water each time (before, during, and after) you exercise. On the days that you exercise, you will probably drink more than the recommended daily amount. As mentioned earlier, it's a nice incentive for each family member to have a new water bottle.

When exercising, avoid drinks with caffeine, which will dehydrate you. This includes tea, coffee, and sodas such as Coke and Mountain Dew. Worse still are drinks with sugar; in addition to sodas, this includes sugary sports drinks marketed as thirst quenchers, such as PowerAde. You only need sports drinks that replace electrolytes or offer other nutrients if you exercise at a steady rate for longer than an hour—otherwise, plain water will suffice. If you find plain water boring, you can add lemon, lime, or orange slices, and pour it over ice.

Activity 3: Body Image

Bodies come in all different shapes and sizes. People have different metabolisms, bone structures, genes, habits, and taste buds. We also have very different ways of seeing ourselves, and unique personal ways of reacting to what we see when we look in the mirror. A beautiful woman can look at her reflection and see only her flaws. A short fat bald man can see an attractive Hollywood movie star in the mirror. We don't always see ourselves as we really are.

Take some time and write the answers to the questions in the Body Image Survey, which should be in everyone's folder (see page 241).

Discuss why it's important to establish body pride. Body image and self-esteem are connected. Having a negative opinion about your body can have a negative impact on your ego, and without body pride, people tend to make less of an effort to eat healthily and exercise. People sometimes hang on to their weight as a way to cope with anger or fear.

Having pride in your body is a skill you can develop. Previously, you may have told yourself, "I'm too fat." But you can learn to say, "I am becoming stronger and healthier." It takes courage, and often you have to leap before you feel you're ready: participating in sports, going to the beach, or to a party before you think you're "thin enough." You can respect your body the way it is. The more self-respect you have, the less likely you are to overeat.

Ask yourself, "What does my body say to other people?"

Some people use their overweight bodies to speak for them without using words. What that is exactly varies from person to person. One child might be saying to a critical parent, "You can't control me." Another who is afraid of making friends or who feels terribly shy might be saying to the kids at school, "Stay away from me—I don't want you to know me." Another person might hold on to their weight as a way of saying, "You can't push me around—my size gives me power."

What are other ways of saying those things? How would you say those things with words? What's another way of telling a critical parent, "You can't control me?" What's another way of using words to tell someone, "I'm feeling shy and awkward and I'm afraid if you get to know me you won't like me and I'll feel hurt?" What's another way of saying, "You can't push me around?"

You can lose weight without changing any of the good things about yourself. Changing your weight means changing your health, and changing your health means changing your destiny, for the better. You can set limits, start small, gain self-control, reach your goals, and learn how to take care of yourself. Accepting your body will become a powerful thing, and it will help you feel in control.

In the end, everyone has a lot of good qualities. If we focus on only our imperfections, we aren't really seeing ourselves anymore. What are your positive qualities? Do your have attractive eyes? Strong hands? Are you unbeatable at checkers? Whatever your qualities are, they are what make you unique.

"KidShape is a safe environment for children to discuss their feelings regarding the issues of food and weight."

—KidShape parent

Activity 4: Review Your Trip to the Supermarket

This is the time to review the homework assignment from the last workshop—going to the supermarket and choosing healthy foods. Discuss the following questions:

1. What items did you select?

2. Did you try anything new?

3. What foods do you usually buy? How do they look to you now?

10,000 Steps

You've probably heard of 12-step programs, but did you know there's a 10,000-step program that could help you lose weight?

No, it's not an extremely complicated process in 10,000 parts, but rather a fitness regimen that originated in Japan and has been examined in many subsequent clinical studies, in which participants were encouraged to walk 10,000 steps (a distance of approximately five miles) in the course of a day as they completed simple household tasks. And no, you don't have to keep a running total in your head as you go about your daily business. All you need is a simple digital pedometer, available at any sporting goods store for as little as $15, and a good pair of walking shoes.

What doctors at the Wakayama Medical College discovered was that people who put at least 10,000 steps on their pedometers each day over a 12-week period showed profound improvements in their health, including lower blood pressure and increased exercise capacity, while burning an extra 2,000 to 3,500 calories per week. This study was published in 2000, and since then 10,000-step programs have been endorsed by the U.S. surgeon general and adopted by a variety of schools, clubs, HMOs, and local government agencies throughout the country.

You can try this approach in your family. Start by purchasing pedometers for everyone. Let your kids wear one for a few days, just to get a sense of their starting points. A normal, physically fit child will already fall in the 12,000- to15,000-step range. People considered sedentary walk between 4,000 and 6,000 steps a day, while true couch potatoes log only 2,000 to 4,000 steps per day.

Once you know where you're starting from, you can make a plan to get in at least 10,000 steps daily. That can mean walking with your kids, in parks or on treadmills, or it can mean simply adjusting the way you go about your ordinary business. If you go to the supermarket, park at the far end of the parking lot. If you go to the mall, park at the opposite end from the store you want to go to. Inside the mall, avoid elevators and escalators and take the stairs. For parents, if you work in an office building, use the stairs instead of the elevators, and if you have to talk to someone, take a stroll to your colleague's office instead of using the telephone or e-mail. Use the coffee machine or restroom farthest from your office. Parents or kids who work on computers should get up and walk around every 30 minutes. In the home, try to think of ways to keep moving when you might otherwise sit still. If you're brushing your teeth or talking on the phone, do it while you're walking around. If you're vacuuming, try doing it at a faster pace. Mow the lawn once a week instead of every two weeks, or use a rake instead of a leaf blower. Take the batteries out of all your remote controls so that you have to actually get up to change the channel.

Of course, you have already made a commitment to increase your activity by participating in vigorous exercise for at least 30 minutes, three times a week. The beauty of using a pedometer throughout the day is that it allows you to measure both your vigorous activity and routine activity. These should both be counted toward your 10,000-steps. (For vigorous activities that cannot be measured using a pedometer, such as swimming, biking, or rowing, just keep track of the time, and make allowances for that activity in your step total for that day.) The important thing to remember is that the small things matter, because small things add up to big changes. And by making some simple changes, you will soon see how easy it is to get to 10,000 steps. Every journey begins with a single step.

Weekly Goals

On your Weekly Goals form, fill in the following goals:

1. I will drink six glasses of water per day.

2. I will eat a healthy snack from the Healthy Snack list (pages 82–83).

3. I will practice a new exercise (_____) that I can do by myself (see Exercises to Do by Yourself on pages 166–167).

4. I will do a new physical activity with my family (see Group Activities on pages 162–166).

Homework Assignment

Continue to update your Weekly Food Log, Weekly Activity Log, Weekly Journal Page, and Weekly Goals.

To prepare for the next workshop, write down a list of your four favorite restaurants and what you like about them: the food, the location, the décor, the people who work there. Can you remember your favorite time in a restaurant?

You should continue to eat together as a family at least five times a week and exercise together at least three times a week for 30 minutes.

Possible Journal Topics

Read these topics aloud so everyone can choose what to discuss in their Weekly Journal Pages.

1. How do I feel before I exercise?

2. How do I feel during the time I'm exercising?

3. How do I feel after I exercise?

4. What reasons do I give not to exercise?

5. What would make it easier to get regular exercise?

6. What kind of body do I want to have, and what are the small steps I need to take to get to where I want to be?

7. Who can help me when I'm having trouble exercising?

WHAT PARENTS SHOULD KNOW

Becoming physically active for a sedentary child is a huge change—so take steps to make it as much fun as possible. The American Dietetic Association suggests several ways you can support your child's transition into an active, healthy child.

Be physically supportive. *That means finding activity classes your child might enjoy, driving them there and back, making sure they have the proper clothing, and attending games and performances.*

Encourage participation in sports. *Find a sport appealing to your child. Some kids like team sports while others prefer individual sports such as swimming, tennis, or dance.*

Give positive reinforcements. *Never criticize your child's performance, and praise kids for their participation. Make sports enjoyable and fun for them, and reward their enthusiasm (but not with food).*

Celebrate special occasions with physical fitness. *For your child's birthday, give fitness equipment like a bike or a skateboard to encourage active play, rather than a video, which promotes passive behavior. For birthday parties, take kids to bowling alleys or skating rinks, rather than the movies.*

Make exercise routine. *You can blend activity into your daily life by pushing a lawn mower instead of riding one, taking the stairs instead of the elevator, or walking to the store instead of driving.*

Plan family outings. *You can take the whole family places on weekends to hike, swim, bike, hit golf balls, or do other activities.*

Limit television and computer or video games. *Kids should learn to keep idle activities in proportion. With limits in place, kids will think of something else to do.*

Show them how to do it. *You are your children's role model. If you exercise for 30 minutes a day, they'll see exercise as a natural part of a normal day.*

Volunteer. *After-school programs that promote fitness and sports teams can always use help.*

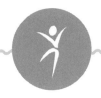

CHAPTER 9

WORKSHOP 5
Eating Out at Restaurants

The primary goal of this workshop is to develop reliable strategies so that you can enjoy eating out at restaurants without sabotaging all the positive steps you've already taken.

Review what you talked about at the last meeting and ask if anybody has any questions, or if there's anything anybody wants to go over. People should share the things they've written in their Weekly Journal Pages if they want to.

Once again, add up the points you've earned on your Weekly Point Charts and record them on the Family Reward Chart. Ask if anybody wants to cash in their points, or if they'd rather keep working toward something larger.

Then read aloud from the following:

A Restaurant Is Not a Health Spa

Jonah, 12, often ate in restaurants. When he came into his doctor's office, he was 64 inches tall and weighed 175 pounds, with a BMI of 30, well above the 95th percentile. He also had high blood pressure and high cholesterol.

His mother, Caroline, was a successful real estate agent in Beverly Hills. Her life was filled with meetings, house showings, and late-night closings for properties in Los Angeles's "Golden Triangle" of Beverly Hills, Bel Air, and Brentwood. She never intended to put her career ahead of her child, but as her marriage crumbled, she had to work. When Jonah was younger, she left him with a sitter, but felt guilty about it. Now she paid the housekeeper extra to look after him when he came home from school. Before the divorce, her husband, Jerry, a well-known entertainment lawyer, would pitch in, but now she had Jonah alone four days a week and every other weekend. Her friends told her they admired her and thought she was a "superwoman," but she knew different. There was literally no time to get everything done, and no time to prepare meals. To compensate, on the four nights a week that Jonah was at Caroline's house, she would race home from the office, pick him up, and tell him he could choose any place he wanted to eat out—no limit.

Jonah's father, Jerry, who'd never been much of a cook, had a similar approach when he had Jonah. Both parents were in a sense trying to impress and win over their son with food. Jerry and Jonah would dine out or order takeout, rent a movie, and eat in front of the television. In addition, Jonah's substantial allowance let him buy anything he wanted. Often, on the way home from school, he'd stop and pick up a 64-ounce Big Gulp to drink while he did his homework.

It wasn't hard to figure out where Jonah was getting all the extra calories, nor to understand the emotional reasons why he might eat more than he needed.

Now Caroline made (and kept) a vow to be home for dinner and to cook as many healthy meals as she could. She also turned off her cell phone for two hours in the evenings and gave her son her full attention, something he'd been craving. Jonah learned to eat smaller portions those nights when his parents took him to restaurants. Caroline exercised with Jonah three times a week and more when she could. In a year, Jonah had grown six inches and lost 13 pounds, and his BMI was a more normal 23.3. His blood pressure and his cholesterol were normal as well. In the end, Caroline lost 35 pounds herself.

We do love to eat out.

On special occasions, birthdays, holidays, anniversaries, romantic dates, get-togethers with friends, or simply when we're alone and need to cheer ourselves up, we go out to eat rather than stay home and prepare something special. Why go to all the trouble of preparing a meal and cleaning up when we can get something that tastes better for nearly the same amount of money and none of the fuss? Or we eat out because we're in too much of a hurry, or had to work late, or have more work to do when we get home. So we pick up a bag of food from one of the thousands of fast-food franchises waiting to serve us.

We are all eating more junk food than we used to. According to a USDA bulletin, the number of calories consumed from fast-food restaurants quadrupled from 1977 to 1996. More people than ever before are eating in restaurants of all kinds: The *Mastercard Dining Out Survey* reported that 46 cents of every dollar we spend on food is now spent on food eaten outside the home, nearly double from 50 years ago.

And restaurants make a business of giving us more calories than we need. Steak houses serve up slabs of prime rib big enough to choke a grizzly bear. Mexican restaurants offer burritos nearly the size of footballs. Breakfast places sell pancakes an inch thick and bigger than the plates they come on (which are also bigger than they used to be) and stack them three or five high. People think big servings are a good deal, so restaurants serve us more than we need. And when more food is sitting in front of us, we eat more. The *Mastercard Dining Out Survey* found that if the food in restaurants were prepared and served the same way we eat at home (that is, smaller portions with less fat) we'd consume nearly 200 fewer calories per day, the equivalent of about 18 extra pounds of body fat per year.

Restaurants compete with each other for that 46 cents of our food dollar by offering a combination of quality, quantity, price, and atmosphere—not by offering food that's good for us to eat. Even the salads at fast-food restaurants feature high-calorie ingredients that tempt us: cheese, croutons, bacon bits, and dressing.

It feels special to eat in a restaurant where, unlike at home, you can order what you want or request how you want your food prepared. You don't have to have the same salad dressing as everybody else, or the same vegetables, and you can have your own special dessert.

Parents, of course, drive the car and choose the restaurant—and many are guilty of saying, "Order anything you want." Parents might try to steer their children clear of giant "value" meals that contain close to 2,000 calories, but the child probably still ends up with a fried, fatty meal with a sugary drink and maybe dessert as well.

Eating out in a restaurant should be special—but there are right ways and wrong ways to eat out. Most restaurants will, for example, change your order if asked, putting dressing on the side, broiling instead of frying, and so on. Some will bring half orders, or let you share meals. Frequently appetizers are large enough to eat as a regular portion. Even at fast-food restaurants, you can make wise choices, choosing plain side salads, chili, baked potatoes, or small hamburgers instead of giant orders of fries and burgers. By paying attention to fat and sugar contents and portion sizes, we can still eat healthily and happily in restaurants.

You can still "have it your way," in any restaurant you go to. And if a restaurant refuses to give you the food you want, the way you want it, well, there are always other restaurants. And if Grandpa seems disappointed when you don't order seconds or refills or dessert, it's all right—he will eventually understand.

Check-in

Begin by discussing what happens to you emotionally when eating out at a restaurant, where temptations abound and you cannot control what's available to eat. Count up how many times in the past week you ate meals that were not prepared at home, including pizzas you picked up or had delivered, as well as food picked up at drive-through windows. Many people are surprised to discover that they eat out more than they think.

What kinds of foods do you eat when you eat out? Do you look for the biggest or richest item, because you want to get the most for your money? Do you splurge on rich foods that you wouldn't ordinarily eat, because it is a once-in-a-blue-moon sort of occasion?

What prevents you from eating at home? Do you feel like you never have the time (even though a grilled turkey burger, steamed vegetables, and a salad could take as little as 20 minutes to put together with everybody helping—if you had thought ahead to buy the ingredients)?

Survival Guide to Fast Food

Everyone knows that many fast foods are high in fat and calories. Obviously, the best strategy is to avoid fast-food restaurants. But fast-food restaurants are everywhere, and sometimes they are hard to avoid. For a convenient guide to the calories and fat in many popular fast-food selections, use the Carry-Along Fast-Food Guide Tables on pages 247–248. You can tear these out of the book (or photocopy them, or print them from www.kidshape.com) and keep them in your purse, wallet, or glove compartment. In addition, here are some tips for cutting the fat in your fast food:

→ Hold the mayonnaise and other dressings that are high in fat, like the special sauce on the Big Mac. If you order a Double Whopper with Cheese without mayonnaise, the fat grams go from a whopping 63 fat grams to 43 grams.

→ Choose grilled, charbroiled, or baked foods, not fried.

→ Drink 1 percent fat milk, nonfat milk, unsweetened iced tea, or water instead of soda.

→ Use less dressing on salad and choose reduced-fat or fat-free dressing. Also, stay away from higher-fat toppings like avocado, bacon bits, deep-fried croutons, eggs, olives, and sunflower seeds.

→ Remove skin and breading from chicken.

→ Order small fries instead of large, and share with your family.

→ Choose a regular burger instead of a specialty burger.

→ Choose a turkey or roast beef deli sandwich.

→ Make your baked potato lean by topping with salsa, mustard, beans, or broccoli.

Activity 1: Restaurant Role-Playing

What ways can you think of, when eating in restaurants, to reduce the portion size or calorie and fat content of the dishes you order?

Give it a try through role-playing.

Somebody pretends to be a server (waiter, waitress, or drive-up window clerk). One or more of the family members pretends to be ordering in a restaurant. As each person orders a meal from an imaginary menu (keep it realistic, modeled on the kinds of restaurants you like to go to), the server should write that person's order down, along with the name of the person ordering. Try to order as healthy a meal as you can.

Then, one by one, look at each person's meal. Does it resemble the food pyramid or their personal food plan? Look at each item ordered and see if there's a way to improve it. If you ordered a salad, what kind of dressing did you ask for: regular or low fat? If you ordered meat, did you ask for it broiled or fried? What would you do if there is nothing healthy on the children's menu? (Answer: Order a healthy adult meal, eat half, and take half home as leftovers.) What would you do if somebody unconcerned about diet orders an unhealthy appetizer for the whole table? (Answer: If you really want some, have a piece but skip your bedtime snack, or if you have more than a small taste, plan to allow time for extra exercise tomorrow.)

Use the restaurant tips in Table 9.1 to help you. You should also review the Survival Guide to Fast Food on page 129.

Now try again. Have someone else pretend to be the server, but go around again and practice ordering healthy meals.

Did you do better?

Activity 2: Review Your Favorite Restaurants

Review last week's homework assignment. Go over your favorite restaurants. For a family of four, there may be as many as 16 restaurants, so choose the top five to discuss. For each restaurant, answer the following questions together. The leader should make written notes.

RESTAURANT TIPS

MENU ITEMS	FOODS TO ENJOY	FOODS TO LIMIT
Appetizers	Clear soups, such as broth, fresh fruit, fish cocktail, steamed or raw vegetable platter, garden salad.	Creamed soups, fried or breaded vegetables, creamy salad dressings, any other fried items.
Entrées	Baked, broiled, boiled, grilled, charbroiled, roasted, blackened, barbequed.	Fried, sautéed, marinated, breaded, stuffed, creamed.
Vegetables	Stewed, steamed, boiled, fresh, baked.	Au gratin, creamed, fried, escalloped, sautéed.
Salads	Tossed vegetable salads with low-fat dressing or dressing on the side, fruit salad.	Mixed salads made with mayonnaise, creamy dressing, added cheese.
Breads	Sliced breads, rolls, baguettes, crackers.	Garlic bread, cheese bread.
Fats	None, or oil and vinegar dressing.	Margarine, cream, butter, sour cream, bacon.
Desserts	Fresh fruit, sorbet, sherbet, angel food cake, gelatin.	Cakes, pies, mousse, puddings, ice cream, cookies.
Drinks	Water, juice and water mixed (50/50), low-fat or nonfat milk, unsweetened iced tea, diet soda (drink diet soda only occasionally).	Regular milk, malts, milkshakes, regular sodas, fruit-flavored drinks.

TABLE 9.1

1. What is the name of the restaurant?

2. What is your favorite item on the menu? Is it healthy? Why or why not?

3. What could you do to make it healthier?

4. What would be healthier choices?

Keep your notes with you for the next time you go out to eat, so that you can practice.

Activity 3: A Test Run

This exercise can't be done in the home. It's time to go to a real restaurant (avoid fast-food restaurants the first time, though you may want to try one the second time) and put to use the things you've been learning. Be sure to bring with you any written notes you made about the restaurant in the previous activity. As you look at the menu, try to identify items that are low in fat or healthy. Try to identify ways to modify the foods you want to make them healthier.

"The best subjects we covered were restaurants, portion sizes, and how to read a label."

—KidShape parent

When the server comes, be polite but order your food exactly the way you want it. Let kids know there's nothing wrong with telling the server you're on a diet and have some special needs. Practice placing limits on yourself. When everyone orders, refrain from commenting or correcting, but pay compliments afterward for good decisions. Make sure when the food arrives that it's been prepared the way you asked. If it hasn't, teach kids how to send their food back politely so that the chef can correct the mistake. Teach them as well to be complimentary to the staff and leave a good tip if the food is delicious and well prepared.

Use Table 9.2 for a guide to selecting healthy foods in ethnic restaurants. See also Table 9.3 for a general guide to the calories and fat in some typical foods in ethnic restaurants.

ETHNIC RESTAURANT LOW-FAT FOOD CHOOICES

TYPE OF FOOD	CHOOSE MORE OFTEN	CHOOSE LESS OFTEN
Chinese	Steamed or lightly stir-fried chicken, fish, lean meat, rice, or vegetables. Mix one cup entrée with one cup steamed rice or steamed vegetables to dilute the sauce.	Fried entrées, fried rice, fried wonton, fried noodles, Peking duck, pork, spare ribs.
Italian	Pasta with marinara sauce, vegetarian pizza with little or no cheese.	Pasta with butter, cream, Alfredo, cheese, meat, and pesto sauce; lasagna; eggplant or veal parmesan; Caesar salad; sausage, pepperoni, or cheese pizza.
Mexican	Chicken, fish, lean meat, beans and vegetables cooked without adding oils, bean burrito or enchilada without cheese, salsa, corn tortillas.	Regular burritos, tacos, enchiladas, chile rellenos, refried beans, guacamole and sour cream, cheese, corn chips, nachos.
Southern	Baked chicken, fish and potatoes, boiled greens, black-eyed peas, sweet potatoes, beans—cooked with turkey instead of ham hocks, grits (without butter or cheese), gumbo, and jambalaya.	Fried chicken, ham, bacon, sausage, chitterlings, corn bread, biscuits, peach cobbler, butter pound cake.
Japanese	Blackened fish, grilled chicken, fish or lean meat, sushi, sashimi.	Seafood or vegetable tempura, teriyaki beef or chicken.

TABLE 9.2

GENERAL RESTAURANT NUTRITION FACTS

CHINESE FOOD

Food item	Calories	Fat grams	% calories from fat
Almond cookie	45	3	60%
Cashew chicken	230	14	39%
Chow mein, chicken	255	10	35%
Egg roll, 1	180	10	50%
Rice, fried, 1 c.	376	10	24%
Rice, white, 1 c.	162	trace	0%
Sweet and sour shrimp	953	84	79%
Vegetable stir fry	85	trace	0%

ITALIAN FOOD

Food item	Calories	Fat grams	% calories from fat
Beef ravioli	220	5	18%
Chicken cacciatore	220	8	33%
Cheese ravioli	415	17	37%
Fettuccini Alfredo	432	30	63%
Garlic toast, 1 slice	121	4	29%
Lasagna with meat, 8 oz.	305	11	33%
Minestrone soup	82	2	27%
Spaghetti with meatballs, 8 oz.	241	10	37%

MEXICAN FOOD

Food item	Calories	Fat grams	% calories from fat
Bean burrito, 1	387	14	32%
Beans, frijoles, 1 c.	225	8	32%
Beef burrito, 1	431	21	44%
Beef taco, 1	370	21	51%
Beef tamales, 2	224	16	64%
Chicken fajitas, 2	520	8	14%
Chorizo, 1 link	273	23	76%
Enchilada, cheese, 1	320	19	53%
Refried beans, 1 c.	248	2	7%
Spanish rice, 1 c.	213	4	17%
Taco salad	660	37	50%
Tortilla chips, 1 oz.	136	7	46%

TABLE 9.3

Weekly Goals

On your Weekly Goals form, fill in the following goals:

1. I will plan and prepare (with adult help, as necessary) a healthy meal at home (see recipes on pages 178–204).

2. I will use measuring cups to measure out correct portions of foods.

3. I will practice stretches (see pages 170–176).

4. I will take a 30-minute walk with a family member.

Homework Assignment

Keep track of your eating, exercise, and feelings in your Weekly Food Log, Weekly Activity Log, and Weekly Journal Page. Continue to monitor your progress on your Weekly Goals chart.

To prepare for the next workshop, make a list of all the foods you like to eat at special occasions such as Thanksgiving, Christmas, or birthdays. Design two menus, one the most decadent you can think of, the other the healthiest.

As always, you should eat together as a family at least five times a week and exercise together at least three times a week for 30 minutes.

Possible Journal Topics

Everyone should write about restaurants. Read aloud the following questions, so family members can choose which topics they want to discuss in their Weekly Journal Pages.

1. How many times a week do I eat out?

2. If it's a lot, how can I cut back?

3. What are the reasons that I eat out, when I could eat at home?

4. Which restaurants are better than others?

5. How sensible are my choices when I eat out?

6. How can I customize the meals served in restaurants to make them healthier?

WHAT PARENTS NEED TO KNOW

What has become known in recent years as the "Atkins diet" restricts highly refined carbohydrates, such as breads, rice, and potatoes, and replaces them with protein, moderate fat, and limited carbohydrates. Diets like this have been advocated for over a century and have swung in and out of fashion over the years. There's no question that these diets can promote rapid weight loss, when rapid weight loss is needed. Certainly for patients with insulin resistance syndrome, these low-carbohydrate diets are useful and effective.

Some adults, however, who chose to consume large amounts of fatty food such as bacon, whipped cream, and avocados without adhering to the rest of the plan harmed their serum cholesterol and triglyceride levels. Instead of helping cure their problems, they made them worse.

For children, the Atkins diet may present a potentially harmful protein load, leading to impaired kidney function. You should not attempt to eliminate carbohydrates from children's diets. Carbohydrates are a necessary part of a healthy diet because they provide the body with the energy it needs for physical activity and to keep organs functioning properly. What you can do is reduce or eliminate foods with processed carbohydrates and those high in sugar, and instead reach for natural carbohydrates, including starchy vegetables, fruit, and whole-grain oats or bread.

The main concern about any fad diet is that when a person returns to "normal eating," the lost weight returns. So the best plan—especially for children— remains a sensible diet with portion control and a wide variety of foods.

CHAPTER 10

WORKSHOP 6

Dealing with Special Occasions

This workshop will help you make wise choices even when participating in special events, such as birthday parties or holiday meals. While restaurants offer a distraction from healthy eating, parties and other such festive meals can also create powerful temptations.

After adding up the points everyone has earned since last time on the Weekly Point Charts and Family Reward Chart, ask how everybody is feeling. Is exercise getting easier, now that you're getting used to it and your muscles have lost their initial soreness? Does anyone have any new ideas about activities you might want to all do together? Does anyone want to share any thoughts from the Weekly Journal Pages? Or say anything about the support you've been getting from the others? Has anyone been particularly helpful?

Then read aloud from the following:

Holidays Are Not Holidays from Eating Sensibly

The pediatrician told Sandra, a 40-year-old stay-at-home mom, that her daughter, Marta, needed to lose 20 pounds. So twelve-year-old Marta reluctantly attended a weight loss and exercise program. She had just begun to adjust to the new way of thinking about health, diet, and exercise when Sandra foresaw a huge roadblock looming—Thanksgiving.

Sandra was a first-generation American, born in Los Angeles to parents who'd emigrated from Mexico. She'd spoken only Spanish until she went to school, where she was only allowed to speak English. On Thanksgiving Sandra's family consumed many of the usual Thanksgiving foods. However, for Sandra, a large part of hanging on to her heritage involved eating and preparing traditional Mexican foods, from recipes and techniques passed down from her abuela, *Rosa, who was very much the matriarch of the family. Rosa insisted on serving menudo every Sunday, a traditional Mexican dish made with beef tripe (stomach linings) and hominy, and hosting tamale parties where the tamales were made from scratch using hand-ground masa and highly fattening lard. Sandra remembers the parties for the conviviality as much as for the food produced. "We'd all sit around and drink beer and have so much fun," she recalls. Rosa made sure that traditions were upheld. "When I tried to make menudo out of chicken one time instead of beef tripe, she just looked at it and laughed," Sandra says.*

It's hard to give up foods connected emotionally to such positive feelings and memories. It was nevertheless important to Sandra, with a big Thanksgiving feast approaching, to make sure Marta stayed on target and didn't suffer from a significant lapse. When Sandra prepared the stuffing, she used a fat-free squeeze margarine in place of butter, added chicken broth to moisten it, and cooked the stuffing outside the turkey instead of inside it. She served steamed vegetables, lightly coated with zero-calorie butter-flavored spray, and a sweet broccoli salad made with turkey bacon and a dressing of nonfat mayonnaise, vinegar, and honey. In addition to mashed potatoes, she had intended to serve sweet potatoes that were simply baked, rather than candied. However, she was overruled by her oldest son, John, who had recently returned from the war in Iraq and was craving traditional foods. John cooked the sweet potatoes himself, using molasses and brown sugar.

Sandra watched proudly as Marta served herself the correct portions of the foods offered, taking only half a cup of mashed potatoes where in previous years she would have piled her plate high. Marta said "no, thank you" to the buttered rolls an aunt had brought, and made other choices as to which temptations to give in to and which ones weren't worth the extra calories.

"I could see Marta thinking, saying to herself 'that's not worth it' and really limiting herself, without having to be told," reports Sandra. "It would have been nice if everything on the table were absolutely healthy, but you know, that's the real world. Especially at a family meal, where other people bring in dishes you can't control. The trick is knowing your choices, knowing your portions, and making trades."

The turkey was moist and wonderful, the stuffing was a big hit, and everything went well. Best of all, before the feast Sandra organized a family soccer game, adults versus kids, using a large beach ball at a nearby park. Everyone had a chance to run around and "work up an appetite." Of course, what Sandra and Marta and the others were actually doing was burning calories, a good way to prepare for the surfeit of riches to follow. At 87, Rosa refrained from joining in the soccer game, but she ate with everyone else and had a big smile on her face when the feast was over. Marta was smiling too.

"The only thing that didn't work was the gravy," Sandra says. "We bought a can of fat-free gravy at the store instead of making it from the drippings ourselves, and it was not a big hit, even for me. So we'll try something different next year. We'll figure it out."

On holidays it's extremely difficult for kids trying to watch what they eat to stay on course, particularly when everyone else is in the mood to indulge. Grandparents prepare rich, traditional foods. Aunts and uncles enter the house bearing pies and cakes.

By definition, traditions resist change. Our grandparents, great-aunts, and great-uncles grew up in a time of relative nutritional innocence. Little was known of the dangers of the various foods. Food was considered good when it tasted good and filled you up. Back then it was also true that most foods were purchased fresh and didn't yet contain the dyes and preservatives and additives they now contain. Food was to be enjoyed, not worried over.

The family feast is a time when we return to old-fashioned foods and recipes that have been passed down for generations. Every culture has its own traditions and rituals. In America, we eat turkey at Thanksgiving. There's also gravy, stuffing, mashed potatoes, sweet potatoes, corn, green beans, cranberry relish, apple pies, pumpkin pies, pecan pies, and all the unique foods each family adds to the traditional meal, where a hungry person can easily consume an entire day's worth of calories in a single sitting. We eat special foods at Christmas, Passover, Kwanza, or the Chinese New Year. These foods and occasions are sacred to us.

No one should be forbidden from participating in family feasts. They are, in many ways, the finest representations of the family table and a source of strength and pride for all of us. They are the times we remember when we look back on our lives, and they connect us to our past and our heritage.

The key is this: We can eat what we want if we know how to eat it. With a bit of advance preparation, we can still indulge in our favorite holiday foods while exercising the portion-control techniques we learned in previous lessons. One example is Halloween candy. If we know we're allowed a certain amount of sugar per day, we can make sure that the amount of sugar in the Halloween candy we eat is included in our total allowance for the day.

We can also learn how to resist temptation. There are many ways we can say no to family members and friends who are offering unhealthy foods, or to hosts at parties passing hors d'oeuvres around the room.

We are not on a zero-tolerance regimen! We can and should enjoy ourselves during special occasions and family feasts—but we don't have to overdo it. We can taste everything if we remember to keep things in proper proportion. Staying healthy is a better way to celebrate life than overeating.

STOP

Check-in

In some families, and in many cultures, the rituals of feting and feasting are the glue that holds the family unit together. Families partake of celebratory meals where the food is often unhealthful, yet the eating of it is mandatory, lest ethnic or cultural traditions be broken or hosts' feelings be hurt.

What's it like in your home? What Christmases or seders or Thanksgivings do you remember? What do you remember about them? How about other special occasions? Dinner parties, New Year's Eve celebrations, Super Bowl parties, Halloween, graduations, anniversaries, or slumber parties? There are usually all kinds of sweet or fatty things to choose from and very few low-fat options at such occasions. Talk about temptation.

Activity 1: Special Occasions Role-Playing

Act out the following scenarios. Volunteers can choose roles or invent new ones as you improvise. The idea is to come up with solutions to difficult situations. After the "actors" have finished, discuss the possible solutions and mention the suggested possibilities below each scenario.

SITUATION 1: You're at a birthday party, and you've already eaten a cheeseburger, but then the ice cream and cake come out.

Good solutions: Have some and walk or run an extra half hour the next day. Have only a taste. Have some and skip dessert at dinner and your bedtime snack.

SITUATION 2: You've gone trick-or-treating with your friends and have collected a lot of Halloween candy.

Good solutions: Choose your favorites and set them aside. You can incorporate one or two pieces into your daily meal plan if you eliminate some other source of sugar from your diet. You can give away the rest of the candy to a shelter or food pantry. You can always throw the candy away.

SITUATION 3: You're at a big family gathering where there are lots of rich, unhealthy foods to choose from. Relatives are pushing food toward you—what do you do?

Good solutions: Eat a healthy snack before you go so you're not as hungry. Bring some healthy food with you. Say, "Thanks, but I'm on a diet." Don't stand next to the food table. If you eat more than you should, exercise more than usual the next day.

SITUATION 4: You're at a big family gathering with a massive buffet and nobody's watching you.

Good solutions: Keep a low-calorie drink such as water, sparkling water, or diet soda in your hand to keep from eating too much. Serve your own food and keep your portions small. Eat slowly. Be aware of how hungry you are. Ask yourself if you're eating because you're hungry, or just because the food is there. Take small tastes of the richer, fattier foods. Don't sample the desserts until you already feel full.

SITUATION 5: The family feast is over and you know you ate too much.

Good solutions: Don't expect to be perfect all the time. Remember that special occasions don't happen that often. Think about what worked and what didn't. Think about what you can do differently the next time. Increase your exercise the next day or two.

You can also have some fun by switching roles, where the kid pretends to be the parent and the parent pretends to be the kid. You can wear an article of the other's clothing to get into the role, while other family members are silent observers. (Rotate the parts so that everyone gets to be a child, parent, and silent observer.) Then try to imagine how the person whose part you're playing would address the following questions:

1. Why is weight a problem in this family?

2. What is the child's plan for managing that weight?

3. What support would the child like from the parent?

4. What limits will the parents set for themselves?

5. What expectations does the parent have of the child?

Activity 2: Include More Action in Your Celebrations

Everyone should think of fun ways to incorporate exercise, for the whole group, into holidays. Make a list to refer to later. Some of your exercise ideas —such as a hike in the neighborhood before or after the meal—may be expanded versions of things you do on a regular basis. Or perhaps you, along with your friends and extended family, would enjoy a special touch football game, a trip to the skating rink, or running on the beach. In some communities, there are organized races or walking events on Thanksgiving, like the Turkey Trot in Topanga, California, or the Boulevard Bolt in Nashville. Consider participating in such an event as a family. Some local gyms have special hours and special events on holidays to help you "burn the calories" before you sit down to the big feast. Try to find ways in your community.

"I have tried everything, and I recommend KidShape."

—KidShape parent

Next write down ideas for making birthday celebrations more active. You and your guests might enjoy a birthday party at a playground, swimming pool, bowling alley, YMCA, or ice skating rink. You can even set up active games such as an obstacle course in your backyard or a treasure hunt in your backyard or neighborhood. Keep your lists to refer to when it's time to plan the next party or holiday celebration.

Activity 3: Favorite Holiday Foods

Your homework from the last workshop was to make a list of favorite holiday foods and plan both a decadent and a healthy meal. You should all share your lists of favorite foods. Then discuss the following questions:

1. What kinds of food seem to appear most often on the lists?

2. Why do you think you chose these types of foods? (Possible answers: they are traditional; they are comfort foods.)

3. How can you include these foods in the most healthful way? (Possible answers: limit the portion size; serve or eat them after you have eaten the lighter foods; eat them after you have eaten an apple and had a big glass of water.)

Now share your menus for decadent and healthy meals. What are the differences between the healthy menus and the decadent menus?

Weekly Goals

On your Weekly Goals form, fill in the following goals:

1. I will plan and prepare (with adult help, as necessary) a healthy meal at home (see recipes on pages 178–204).

2. I will make a healthy food choice outside the home.

3. I will measure my pulse rate before and after I exercise.

4. I will do strength-training exercises (see Exercises to Do by Yourself on pages 166–167).

Homework Assignment

As usual, fill in your Weekly Food Log, Weekly Activity Log, Weekly Journal Page, and Weekly Goals.

This week's assignment is to design an awards dinner to celebrate finishing the course, which will be over after the next workshop—although you will, of course, continue healthy eating, regular exercise sessions, and increased daily activities. Kids can help plan the menu and some active party games. You may also want to assign each workshop participant to shop for and prepare one dish (keeping in mind the food guide pyramid). Some dishes may be prepared before the final meeting.

You should each prepare a speech for the awards dinner, to address successes and continued challenges, goals that have been met, and how you feel about the lifestyle changes you've made, both individually and as a family. If you feel a sense of pride, talk about it. Your speech is also a chance to be honest with yourself and others about your lapses.

Also, remember to eat together as a family at least five times a week and exercise together at least three times a week for 30 minutes.

Possible Journal Topics

Read aloud the following questions, which family members can write about in their Weekly Journal Pages.

1. Where did the idea of "the Clean Plate Club" come from? Why is it a bad idea?

2. Why is resisting temptation so difficult? What makes it easier?

3. How can I avoid being pressured into eating too much?

4. Who puts the most pressure on me?

5. What holiday foods do I find the most tempting?

6. Why do we feel we have to eat more than we need during the holidays?

7. Among all the foods at the holiday meal, which ones are better than others?

8. What other ways are there to celebrate that don't use food?

9. What sorts of trade-offs can I make to prepare for a feast?

10. What practical things can I do to avoid the temptation of holiday food?

WHAT PARENTS SHOULD KNOW

- *Food companies spend $12 billion a year marketing their products to children, who see about 40,000 commercials annually, report Michael Jacobson, PhD, and Bruce Maxwell in their book,* What Are We Feeding Our Kids?

- *Studies published in the* Journal of Consulting Clinical Psychology *have shown that obese children who were advised to control their appetites did so—and lost weight.*

- *During the last 30 years, the amount of soda children drink has doubled— and the amount of milk consumed has decreased by half, according to a study in the* Journal of the American Dietetic Association.

- *A child with one overweight parent has a 40 percent chance of being overweight, according to the book* Obesity, *by Per Bjorntorp, MD, PhD, and Bernard N Brodoff, MD. When both parents are overweight, the odds increase to 80 percent.*

- *While sitting still in a chair watching TV, a child's (and an adult's) metabolic rate is 50 percent slower than when just sitting and not watching TV, finds a study published in the* Archives of Family Medicine.

- *Identical twins raised in separate households have similar body types, according to a study reported in the* New England Journal of Medicine, *but a twin raised in a home with poor eating or exercise habits is almost always heavier than the twin raised with good eating habits.*

Chapter 11

WORKSHOP 7
Environmental Self-defense

The primary goal of this workshop is to find ways to integrate what you've learned into family life, both now and in the future.

First, review how many points everyone has earned, adding up the points on everyone's Weekly Point Charts and tallying them on the Family Reward Chart. Then discuss rewards. You may want to continue the reward system indefinitely, or you may want to limit the time during which everyone can work toward the rewards you designated earlier. As always, see if any family members want to share anything from their Weekly Journal Pages.

The final workshop is by no means the last time you'll gather as a group at the family table—eating together is the single most effective tool you'll have to maintain the benefits of the program. Preventing new weight gain is easier than overcoming weight that one has already gained. The workshops in the program are both preventative and remedial. Any one of them can be revisited at any time to refresh the family awareness. It's important that parents continue to spend active time with their children, continually reinforcing the gains each family member has made. Parents need to continue to pay close attention not only to what their children are eating, but also to their moods, activities, social lives, and school performance. The best way to do this is to make sure that the conversation at the family table flows freely and frequently, reinforcing the idea that the joy of eating should come not from what you eat but whom you eat with.

READ-ALOUD FOOD FOR THOUGHT

Finding Your Source of Strength

Ever since she could remember, Jessica had been overweight. She felt there was something wrong with her, because her brother was normal weight and her sister was downright skinny. Her weight made her antisocial. When the kids at school or in the neighborhood teased her or refused to play with her, she told herself she didn't need friends, and had better things to do than play with people.

One day, when Jessica was 13, her mother, Anne, knocked on her bedroom door and told her she was really concerned about her weight.

"I don't care," Jessica said. "Just leave me alone."

In desperation, Anne got angry and told Jessica she wasn't going to let her get away with it. She tried to force Jessica to eat better, cooking low-fat foods and serving smaller portions. She tried to force Jessica to exercise as well, until a little war developed. Jessica decided she hated her mom, and she hated herself too. She felt hungry when she didn't eat and guilty when she did, sneaking food and eating it in hiding. When she tried to exercise (at her mother's insistence) she felt embarrassed and incompetent. She withdrew even further, spending long hours in her room, even though she hated being alone because it left her to deal with her unwanted thoughts. Anne's methods weren't just not working—they were making Jessica feel worse. Anne was acting in anger and frustration, rather than showing Jessica that she was caring and supportive.

Then, on Jessica's 17th birthday, her mother gave her what she called a "soul box." It was a painted wooden box, about the size of a large book, and inside was a compass, a rock, and a few note pads.

"The rock symbolizes stability and strength in your life," Anne explained. "The compass symbolizes the direction you need to take to find yourself." She handed Jessica one of the small note pads. "This is a place for you to write down

whatever makes you feel bad during the day. I want you to write it down and then rip it up and throw it away and be done with it."

Jessica had her doubts and was defiant at first, unwilling to touch the soul box. Gradually, she discovered that when she wrote down the things that made her feel bad and threw them away, she didn't feel so bad any more. Writing them down and throwing them away seemed to clear away her bad feelings. She stared at the rock and knew there was something permanent and good about her, no matter what she looked like. Holding the compass in her hand, she understood that there was a path she was on, and that she would find her way, however many wrong turns she took.

The soul box gave her the will to go to the gym. In five months, she lost 20 pounds and dropped six dress sizes. More significantly, she felt like she could do anything she set her mind to. She opened up and started to talk to people. She made a point of befriending other kids who were overweight, and found that they were happy to share themselves with her. She realized that the strength she needed to lose weight was inside of her all along, as was the ability to feel good about herself. Her spirit had changed, and her body had followed.

Achieving our weight loss goals will be a moment to be applauded and celebrated. It is clearly a difficult thing to do, requiring fortitude and perseverance, and should be acknowledged. Yet it is only one moment. We'll need to be strong because there will be other moments when we may feel tempted or weak.

We are doing more than simply dropping weight before a big party or to fit into our bathing suits during vacation, or even to stop kids from teasing us at school. We are beginning something much more important than that. We are beginning a whole new life of healthy habits by becoming educated about nutrition and exercise. As important as it is, the weight loss itself is not the ultimate goal. More important are the improvements we feel in energy, stamina, and mood. As with Jessica and her soul box, we are rediscovering our inner strengths and becoming reacquainted with our truer selves, the part of us that wants to run and jump and play and feel strong. That's the feeling we want to last a lifetime, a feeling made even better when we can all feel it together as a family.

It's an ongoing process that doesn't end once we've reached our desired weight. We still need limit setting, communication, awareness, and the continued participation of the whole family. It's often after we reach our goals that we have to be the most vigilant, because that's the time when it's entirely human to think, "All right, I've lost 20 pounds—I've suffered and I've earned the right to indulge myself a little bit." Grown-ups who have ridden the roller coaster of cyclical dieting—losing weight, gaining it back and then losing it again—understand how indulging yourself "just a little bit" can too often turn into indulging yourself regularly. Kids need time to develop a sense of impulse control. Over time, reinforcing the idea that the changes made during the program are permanent and not temporary will make it easier and easier for kids to keep on track, but they need their parents' help.

It's worth repeating that none of us is perfect, and we can expect an occasional relapse. Even the most enthusiastic person may return to old habits of overeating and inactivity because of inattention, increased stress, prolonged holidays, or a physical illness that forces a "time out" from activity. In children and teens, relapsing may also result from anger or rebellion against parental expectations, or from a need to control their own lives. The family table, where we have practiced open communication and active listening, remains the best place to deal with the occasional (and normal) setbacks and adjustments.

It's also the best place to recognize when rebellious behavior is a sign of a more serious problem. Most families find that the more kids feel they're being heard and understood, with their opinions taken into consideration, the less angry they feel. When we do feel that way, we can redirect those emotions toward behaviors that aren't self-destructive. We can be healthy and still be ourselves. We can be artists or rock stars, scientists or social workers, restaurant workers or mechanics, or anything we want, but in none of those occupations is it an advantage to be unhealthy or overweight. Whoever we want to be, we can still be fit. It's good when teenagers want to set their own goals and regulate their own progress. And children who learn to set goals when they're young find it easier to set goals as teenagers. Setting goals and making changes is always easier when we have the family table as a resource we can turn to for advice and support.

Maintaining weight loss will require adopting a strategy of "environmental self-defense" to protect ourselves from social messages that try to push us back toward old unhealthy habits. In the real world, we face the daily temptations of fast food, junk food, television, and other passive forms of recreation. We are susceptible to peer pressure, unwilling to be labeled different, or to let on that we have a "problem" with food when the other kids don't. Nobody wants to stand out from the crowd, particularly when the crowd is at McDonald's, chowing down on burgers, fries, and shakes after a soccer game.

Children are also acutely susceptible to the subtle yet powerful messages of advertising. Kids have a better chance of resisting when they are armed early with the knowledge of how to judge portion sizes, how to evaluate whether foods are healthy, and how to select healthy meals in restaurants.

Environmental self-defense simply means incorporating everything we've learned into our daily lives, permanently, from this day forward. It means putting into practice the skills we've learned, such as reading labels and measuring portions, and the techniques we've practiced, such as role-playing and analyzing our feelings about food. Our bodies represent how we live. If we live healthfully and enjoy the natural exuberance that comes from feeling fit and well, our bodies will express that. Diets that concentrate only on weight loss invite the inevitable roller coaster effect of regaining the weight once the dieter is "done." Learning how to practice environmental self-defense will allow us to avoid that roller coaster. It creates a landscape upon which to settle into good habits and behaviors, with a durable and lasting support system firmly in place.

STOP

Check-in

Discuss the importance of environmental self-defense. How can you incorporate what you've learned into your daily lives, to counter all the ways that society and culture might invite you to overindulge? Talk about the full range of real-world eating situations, including birthday parties, office parties, surprise parties, holiday celebrations, social events, play dates and sleepovers, camp, vacations, and family visits.

The key elements of environmental self-defense should include ways to substitute, ways to trade off or work off special occasion foods, ways to make sure the dinner table is a safe and stress-free environment for all of you, and ways to keep open lines of communication between parents and children. Talk about ways to deal with relapses. You are not required to be perfect. You only need to be wiser than you were before. The family should discuss the following questions:

1. What has changed in your life since you started the program?

2. Have the changes been easy or difficult to deal with? Why?

3. What do you think would make the changes easier?

4. Are you surprised at the way you've been able to incorporate healthier choices into your life?

5. What changes are you pleased with, and what would you like to change back?

6. What's the biggest challenge to making changes?

7. What foods do you miss? What's a healthy alternative to those foods?

8. What will you do when you're buying lunch at school or something from a vending machine?

9. What would you do if you were at a friend's house and they offered you an unhealthy snack?

10. Are you surprised at how many unhealthy habits your family had?

Activity 1: Problem Foods

Talk about temptation. Everyone write down all the favorite or problem foods you can think of, the ones you personally have a hard time saying no to. Then on the same line opposite, write down a healthier food you could substitute for each problem food. For example, instead of eating potato chips, your substitute could be low-fat or plain popcorn. Instead of olives, dill pickles. Instead of chocolate, sugar-free chocolate or cocoa. Instead of apple pie, fresh apples. Instead of ice cream, sugar-free low-fat ice cream, sherbet, or sorbet.

What strategies could you develop to keep problem foods at bay?

→ Keep it out of the house—ask your family members not to buy it, and don't buy it yourself.

→ Make it more difficult to eat by keeping it out of sight—put it in the back of the refrigerator, cupboard, pantry or freezer, and wrap it in aluminum foil or a plain brown bag.

→ Keep lower-calorie foods in sight—put the fruit and vegetables and the green snacks up front.

→ Eat from the substitute foods on your list.

→ Do something to take your mind off food—call a friend, go exercise, color or paint, read, go for a walk.

→ Work a small amount into your diet plan (10 potato chips = 1 grain serving + 1 fat serving; 1 small scoop of ice cream = 2 fat servings; 2 small sandwich cookies = 1 grain + 1 fat) and increase your exercise levels afterward.

→ Work off your problem foods. One chocolate chip cookie = 8 minutes of nonstop bike riding; one plain doughnut = 15 minutes of nonstop running; 10 potato chips = 15 minutes of nonstop walking; and so on.

Activity 2: Environmental Self-Defense Role-Playing

Sometimes difficult situations occur in your day-to-day life. But there are always ways to say no to unhealthy choices, and ways to defend yourself against people and situations that sabotage your efforts to stay fit. Act out the following scenarios. After you perform each scene, talk about the solutions the actors devised and discuss the good solutions listed for each scenario.

SITUATION 1: You just finished dinner, but you're still hungry. You're worried your mom will say something if you ask for more food.

Good solutions: Wait 10 minutes to see if you're still hungry. Ask for more vegetables. Have a healthy snack after you clear the dishes.

SITUATION 2: Your sister is selling Girl Scout cookies and your parents buy some to help her out. Thin Mints are your favorite, and there are three boxes sitting on the pantry shelf.

Good solutions: Ask someone to hide them where you can't find them. Limit the amount you have in a day. Ask your parents to give them to a shelter or food pantry.

SITUATION 3: You're staying at your grandparents' house, and they insist that you clean your plate.

Good solutions: Explain to your grandparents that you're on a weight-loss plan. Tell them you want to save the leftovers for lunch tomorrow. Before they serve the food, ask them to give you a smaller helping than usual.

SITUATION 4: You're at a sleepover with friends, and it turns into a royal pig-out, but you're not that hungry.

Good solutions: Eat some, but limit yourself. Pick the healthier snacks: pretzels or baked chips. Eat some of the healthy snacks you brought along (share them with everyone).

SITUATION 5: You had a really bad day at school. You fought with your best friend, failed a math test, and had to stay after school for detention because you forgot your homework. After school, you want to make yourself feel better.

Good solutions: Go for a long run. Take the dog for a walk. Call a friend for support. Hit a punching bag. Talk to your parents.

SITUATION 6: You're in the stall in the restroom at school when you overhear some kids making fun of you.

Good solutions: Leave the stall and say, "Don't you have anything better to do?" Wait for them to leave, take a few deep breaths, and try to let it roll off you. Say from the stall, "I heard that." Confront them later when you've calmed down.

Finally, you can role-play visiting your doctor's office. Kids sometimes have a hard time telling a doctor what it is they're concerned about. Role-playing gives them a chance to practice.

Activity 3: Remeasuring Yourselves

Change into your exercise clothes, if you're not wearing them already, and once again take the fitness test on pages 49–52, repeating the procedures you did when you established your baseline measurements. Record your new results on the Information Survey form (see page 225), which should still be in your folder. Compare them with your earlier results. Remember that the idea is only to compete against yourself and do better than you did the first time you took the test. If you don't improve in certain areas, don't be discouraged. Stay on the path you're on and take the test again in two months, or four, or six.

When you're done, weigh yourselves. Record the date and your weight in the upper left corner on the appropriate chart(s) in your folder [Body Mass Index-for-Age Percentiles (Boys or Girls), Stature-for-Age and Weight-for-Age Percentiles (Boys or Girls), and Body Mass Index Table (Adults); charts are on pages 226–230.] Don't feel bad if you didn't lose much weight: Being able to do more push-ups or sit-ups than before or being able to walk around the block or up a hill or a flight of stairs without getting winded is cause to celebrate. For some of you who are still growing, success will simply mean not gaining any more weight. And the important thing is that you have started a pattern of exercising and eating healthily.

Next measure the height of anyone who might still be growing and then calculate the new BMI, using the formula on page 44 or the automated BMI calculator at www.powerofprevention.com. Write your new BMI down on the chart in your folder [Body Mass Index-for-Age Percentiles (Boys or Girls), Body Mass Index Table (Adults); charts are on pages 226, 228, and 230]. What percentile are you in?

Activity 4: A Personal Reassessment

It's also time to reassess your feelings and attitudes toward food by answering again the questionnaire you filled out when you were first getting started. You should have another copy of Your Personal Food and Fitness Survey in your folder (see page 231).

Now compare the answers you gave the first time you answered these questions with the answers you can give now. What has changed?

Activity 5: A Banquet Just for You

Now it's time for the family to come together to prepare a celebratory feast, the meal you designed as part of last week's homework assignment. Everyone is assigned a job, such as cooking, setting the table, assembling the awards, decorating the room, acting as DJ, or performing as master of ceremonies. Members should dress up.

"KidShape is a safe environment for children to discuss their feelings regarding the issues of food and weight."

—KidShape parent

Talk during dinner about what you've learned. Map out a plan so that each week will include 30 minutes of family exercise at least three times a week. You may want to set goals to increase your level of activity, remembering to take it easy and work up gradually. Discuss ways your kids could join organized teams to get regular physical activity with their peers, either at school or the nearest YMCA or by organizing your own outing clubs for hiking, bird watching, or dog walking, using you as a chaperone if needed.

After dinner, go around the table and announce everybody's point totals and let each participant say how he or she wants to "spend" their points. Parents may share their points with their kids, if they wish.

Then it's time for speeches. Make toasts to all that you've accomplished and to continuing to make healthy choices about eating and exercise. Share with the others the things you've learned about yourselves, and give credit to those who helped push you to achieve your goals. Say thanks and give credit where it's due.

Possible Journal Topics

It's good to keep writing in a journal or in your Weekly Journal Pages (make extra copies if you wish). Kids who overeat often use food to express themselves. Journal writing can give them an alternative way of expressing themselves, and it helps them be honest with themselves about what they're feeling. Your child may benefit from rehearsing in writing what it is he or she wants to say to you before saying it. It's also helpful to reread journal entries if you lose sight of your goals.

You may want to discuss the following in your journals:

1. The end of the program does not mean the end of my new lifestyle. How can I continue applying the things I've learned?

2. What fears do I have about continuing after the workshops end?

3. What was the most surprising lesson I learned?

4. What have I learned about myself that I didn't know before?

5. What would I have done differently?

6. What new goals should I set for myself?

7. What are 10 things I could do to be more active?

8. If I need help reaching those goals, who can I get to help me?

Parents may want to address the following questions in their journals:

1. What things are you or your children doing differently?

2. How are siblings of the overweight child reacting to having less junk food in the house, or having healthier meals?

3. What can you do to make a healthy lifestyle easier for your children?

WHAT PARENTS SHOULD KNOW

- Ø Kids are more easily governed by their impulses and their appetites than grown-ups, and need to be reminded about the lessons they've learned.

- Ø Parents should beware of slipping into old bad habits by including food or television for reward or punishment.

- Ø Children should always be praised for their efforts, and never shamed for their missteps.

- Ø Special care must be taken to distinguish between what children do and who they are—children need to feel loved and accepted for who they are, no matter what they do.

- Ø It's easy to let things slide, and difficult to make changes. Anything your child can do to improve his or her health should be applauded. Children have short attention spans and think in concrete rather than abstract terms, so frequent reminders and reinforcements for even small improvements are required.

- Ø Everyone will progress at a different rate, but any single pound lost is an accomplishment the whole family can take pride in.

- Ø Sometimes you'll be making progress even when you've only stopped gaining weight.

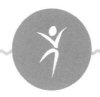

CHAPTER 12

Fun Activities and Sports

We become overweight when we consume more calories than we burn. That statement defines (and clarifies) a problem that we must approach from two angles: nutrition and exercise. Every time you walk a block to mail a letter or lift a heavy dictionary, your muscles use energy your body has consumed or stored. Yet in countless ways, today's obesity epidemic is the predictable result of the technological progress we've seen over the last 100 years, where every invention created to save time or make our lives easier has reduced the number of calories we're required to burn in an average day. A century ago, most of us lived in the country and worked to produce food, plowing fields, pulling stumps, building stone walls, and so on. We did our job only too well—now most of us have moved to the cities, and there's more food than we need and not enough ways to burn calories in the course of an ordinary day. To be fit and healthy, we have to consciously add those activities back into our lives.

Three and 30

Your exercise activities should last a minimum of 30 minutes, and take place three times a week. This is a minimum commitment, though longer or more frequent exercise sessions are allowed. You should begin slowly and work up to your own target heart rate (see pages 116–117). Cut back at the first sign of pain or injury. Remember that there is no hurry, even though it's easy to feel impatient for results. Starting slowly and gradually adding to your exercise program until it becomes a comfortable part of your weekly habit is better than trying to do too much too fast, hurting yourself, and becoming turned off to the process.

While you do want to challenge yourself each time, you needn't push yourself to extremes. Most experts call for "moderately intense" exercise, which can serve as a guideline—go hard, but if things feel too intense, back off. If you're trying to do 50 sit-ups and you can't, don't worry. You'll get there tomorrow, or the next day, or sooner or later. It's not a race, and it's not a competition.

Exercising with Your Dog

Dogs are social animals, descended from the wolf, a predator that hunts in packs, running down larger and faster animals. The dog family has one of the most remarkable cardiovascular systems in the animal kingdom, able to sustain heart rates of over 300 beats per minute for extended periods of time. They love and need to run, and because dogs are social animals, they require our attention and will beg for it in any number of ways.

In a sense, they can show us the way to be fit. Studies have shown that people with dogs as companions tend to live longer and have lower blood pressure, both because dogs give us emotional support and because dogs urge us to exercise. They are always ready and always willing, whatever the weather is like. Their enthusiasm is infectious—our dogs stand at the door wagging their tails as if the walk they're about to take is the best thing that's ever happened to them.

Walking for half an hour a day at a brisk pace will go a long way toward giving you the exercise you need. If you can squeeze in a little Frisbee tossing or tug-of-war with a favorite toy, all the better.

Stretching and Water

You should begin and finish each 3/30 session by stretching (see Chapter 13). The President's Council on Physical Fitness and Sports recommends 10 to 12 minutes of slow stretching daily. You should drink water during exercise, and you should drink at least one eight-ounce glass of water when you're done. The old belief that drinking during workouts should be forbidden has been replaced by the knowledge that frequent rehydration is safer and brings better results.

Water accounts for 60 percent of your body weight and 70 percent of your muscle tissue—you need adequate water to perform at your peak. Water keeps your body cool, evaporating from your skin as sweat when you exercise, which helps cool you off. If you were to put a thermometer in your mouth after a long heavy workout, it would read well over 100 degrees. In the heat of summer, even wearing the lightest of clothing and working out at the coolest times during the day (mornings or evenings), you might lose several pounds of water in a 30-minute workout through sweat, and it's crucial to replace this fluid. If you weigh yourself before and after exercise, drink two cups of water for every pound you've "lost."

"KidShape educates simply, but with great results."

—KidShape parent

In general, drink one to one and a half cups of water 15 minutes before working out, and a cup of water every 10 to 15 minutes during a workout. You should drink water even if you don't feel thirsty, especially if you're outside during the colder months, when you may not be aware of how dehydrated you can get (where winter air is much dryer than summer air). The signs of dehydration include chills, clammy skin, stopping sweating, throbbing heartbeat, and nausea. Signs of more severe dehydration are headaches, cramps, shortness of breath, dizziness, or dry mouth. If such signs occur, stop exercising immediately and drink water, slowly. If the situation doesn't improve, you may wish to seek medical attention.

Group Activities

Any activity that gets your heart pumping is a good activity, but be sure to choose activities in which everyone can participate. From the following varied activities, select as many as you want. The important thing is that you get your metabolism up and that you keep your heart pumping at an optimal level for at least thirty minutes.

CHASE THE FOX. Two people twirl a jump rope. Everyone else plays "follow the fox." The "fox" runs into the rope and does a trick. The trick might be hopping on one foot or touching the ground. Then the fox runs out. Everyone else must repeat the trick. When someone misses, that person becomes a twirler. Continue playing as long as you can.

DANCE. Put the music on and dance. Most communities have organized square dancing, line dancing, contra dancing, and so on. If you're at home, simply clear away the chairs in the dining room and dance there. Kids can pick the music their parents are forced to dance to, and vice versa. You could check out a book or video from the library that teaches a specific dance.

ESKIMO ROLL. Practice somersaults. When you get good, try an Eskimo roll with a partner. Work on a mat or soft grass. Lie on your back with your feet in the air. Your partner stands near your head. Hold on to your partner's ankles as your partner holds yours. Your partner does a somersault. You should end up trading places with your partner. Do this at least three times.

FAMILY OBSTACLE COURSE. Assemble a family obstacle course in the backyard, fixing seven different stations. At station 1, jump rope as fast as you can for 60 seconds. At station 2 (always running between stations), step up and down on a cement cinder block or step for 60 seconds. At station 3, dribble a basketball for 60 seconds. At station 4, do 20 jumping jacks. At station 5, hop on one foot for 30 seconds and then on the other for 30 seconds. At station 6, hula hoop for as long as you can or 60 seconds. At station 7, the last station, complete a

10-yard shuttle run, moving between lines to pick up and retrieve three items, one at a time. You can time each family member if you want. After the first player has moved to station 3, the second player may begin. Depending on how many are playing, fit in as many runs as you can in 30 minutes.

FAST-BREAK BASKETBALL. The game can be played with from one to six children. Use a basketball court or driveway with a basketball hoop at one end, with a marker set up at the other end of the driveway. Players run to the goal, shoot from one to three baskets, then fast-break out to the marker and back to the hoop. Keep shooting until someone steals the ball. Players can use a whiffle ball for variation. Play for 30 minutes.

Kids and Weight Training

Strength training can produce significant results for people trying to lose weight. Strength training creates muscles, and muscles burn calories even when you're at rest. The more muscle mass you have, the more muscle tissue you have burning fat around the clock. Strength training also helps you maintain your lean muscle mass and increases bone density, which helps protect you from injuries.

Kids should not use weights until they're seven or eight years old and can listen to instructions and exercise safely. The idea is never to see how much weight they can lift, but to create an overall benefit. Kids should start with push-ups, pull-ups, and sit-ups, using the body's own weight. They should then move up slowly to light dumbbells, emphasizing upper body exercises.

To begin with, try strength-training sessions twice a week, and give muscles at least 48 hours to rest in between sessions. Exercise physiologist Michael O'Shea, PhD, recommends choosing weights that are comfortable, beginning by doing 5 to 10 different exercises in sets of 8 to 12 repetitions, and working your way up to 10 to 15 repetitions.

FRISBEE. Competitive Frisbee can be played with two to four players to a side. Teams should use a long field with room to run. Two goal lines should be set, one at each end of the field. The object is to try to advance the Frisbee across your opponent's goal line by throwing it to a teammate, who is allowed two steps before throwing to another teammate. If the Frisbee touches the ground, the other team gets possession. If the Frisbee is intercepted or the opponent holding the Frisbee is tagged, the other team gets possession. A team that scores must "kick off" by throwing the Frisbee to the opposing team. The game should be played in two 15-minute halves.

GROUP PULL-UPS. You need four people. Sit on the floor in a circle. Everyone holds hands. Together pull yourselves up to a standing position. Once four of you can do it, add two more to the circle. Experiment on the best way to get up. Do this at least five times.

JUMP ROPE IN THE ROUND. Everyone stands in a circle around one person who is holding a rope with a large knot on the end. The person in the middle twirls the rope in a wide circle close to the ground. Players in the circle must hop over the rope as it passes beneath them. When someone misses, that person becomes the twirler. Repeat until you are exhausted.

LEG WRESTLE. With a partner, lie on your backs with your heads pointing in opposite directions, your knees bent, your legs together, and your feet raised about 18 inches off the ground. Touch the soles of your feet to the soles of your partner's feet. Then push against your partner's feet until one of you can straighten your legs. If you break contact, start over. Repeat until you are exhausted.

SIMON SAYS. This game is best played in a field or park, preferably on a path or trail, but can also be played in the backyard. Players line up in single file and only move when the leader precedes the instructions with the words "Simon Says." If the leader says, "Simon says jump up and down," players jump up and down. If the leader says only, "Jump up and down," anyone who complies must go to the back of the line. The family follows behind the leader in single file along a preset course. Everyone gets a turn to be the leader. Leaders can tell followers to do jumping jacks, hop on one leg, walk backward, quack like a duck while flapping their arms, or anything they think of, as long as it's a physical activity, and as long as "Simon Says."

TAG WITH A TWIST. Try one of these different forms of tag. Play until you are exhausted.

Blackfoot tag. This version was played long ago by Blackfoot Indian children. Form a line with a half dozen people. Hold on to the waist of the person in front of you. The player in front swings the line, trying to turn and tag the person at the end. The person at the end of the line can twist and turn all they want, but must stay attached. When the person at the end is tagged, that person becomes the new front, and the person who was in front moves to the number two position.

Hang tag. You are "safe" as long as you hang by your arms from something, with your feet off the ground. You could hang from a jungle gym or a tree. "It" can tag you only if you are not hanging by your arms.

Hop tag. This version is like regular tag, except that all players must hop on one foot.

Poison tag. As in regular tag, when "It" tags you, you become the new "It." However, you must hold the part of the body where you were tagged with one hand. Keep holding that part of your body until you tag someone else.

Shadow tag. In this variation on regular tag, when the person who is "It" touches your shadow, you become the new "It."

TOE TOUCHES FOR TWO. Lie on the floor head-to-head with a partner so that the tops of your heads are touching. Hold your partner's wrists. Raise your legs until you touch each other's toes. Then return to the starting position. As you get better, increase the distance between your heads. Do this activity as many times as you can.

TUG-OF-PEACE. You'll need about 10 people. Sit in a circle. Place a thick piece of rope inside the circle in front of your feet. Tie the ends of the rope together to make a tight knot. Everyone holds the rope and pulls at the same time. You all should be able to rise to a standing position together. Repeat this activity as many times as you can.

TUG-OF-WAR. Try a two-person tug, using a soccer ball, when one player tries pulling the ball out of the other player's hands. Or using a rope or strong cord, try a one-handed tug-of-war where everyone stands on tiptoes, or a backward tug-of-war where everyone faces away from the middle. Play for as long as the players want to continue. This is a strength-building activity, so the more tired you get, the better.

Exercises to Do by Yourself

There are many exercises you can do when you're by yourself or when there are too few of you to play tag or do other group activities.

PRESIDENT'S COUNCIL ON PHYSICAL FITNESS AND SPORTS CHALLENGE TEST. With the exception of the full curl-ups, you can use the exercises described in Chapter 4 on pages 49–52 as part of your regular exercise regimen.

PUSH-AWAY. Start developing your upper body with the push-away until you can comfortably do three sets of 10 in one workout. Face the wall, standing about three feet away from it or just beyond arm's length. Lean toward the wall, using your arms to stop yourself when your nose is nearly touching the wall. Push yourself back until your arms are fully extended. (Be sure your hands are clean first.)

BENT KNEE PUSH-UP. Once you meet your goal for push-aways, try the bent-knee push-up, Assume the position you would for a regular push-up, but let your knees touch the floor, bending your legs at a right angle.

HANGING LEG RAISES. Hang by your arms from a jungle gym or a pull-up bar mounted on a doorway. Lift your legs up to your waist. Once you can do that, lift your legs up to the bar. Do as many leg raises as you can.

HALF SIT-UPS. Lie on the floor on your back. Your feet are flat. Bend your knees. Fold your arms across your chest. Raise your shoulders so you sit up about halfway. Hold for a couple of seconds. Lie down. Start with two sets of 5 and increase until you can do two sets of 10 in a single workout.

KICKBOARD SWIM: At a pool, a lake, or the beach, hold on to a kickboard with your arms out in front of you. Move yourself by just kicking your legs. Do this for 30 minutes, or at least 10 minutes if you want to combine it with other exercises.

What Different Exercises Can Do

Some exercises are good for building endurance, while others improve your flexibility. In addition, different exercises work different muscle groups. That's why varying your routine is a good idea, and it also helps prevent exercise from becoming boring. There are a wide variety of sports and activities to choose from.

TO IMPROVE AEROBIC CAPACITY (ENDURANCE). Bicycling, swimming, ice skating, roller skating, inline skating, running, jogging, walking, hiking, cross-country skiing, hurdler's jumps, lateral jumps, jumping rope, playing tag, running zig-zags, soccer, full-court basketball, singles racquetball, tennis, badminton, relay races.

TO IMPROVE ABDOMINAL STRENGTH. Bicycling, twirling a hula hoop, hanging leg raises, half sit-ups, swimming without your arms (kickboard swimming), leg wrestling.

TO IMPROVE UPPER ARM STRENGTH. Tennis; volleyball; swinging a baseball bat; throwing a baseball, basketball, or football; tug-of-war; paddling a canoe; group pull-ups; twirling a baton; arm wrestling; swinging from rings.

TO IMPROVE FLEXIBILITY. Gymnastics, tumbling, ballet, dancing, cheerleading, yoga, tae kwon do, karate, other martial arts.

WHAT PARENTS SHOULD KNOW

Your children need your help! This is true both for eating healthfully and for exercising, and it's particularly true when kids are younger. Younger kids are more likely to respond to encouragement from parents and to seek parental approval, where in later years, they look more to coaches, teachers, or peers for reinforcement and support. Younger children also have a strong desire to achieve mastery over physical skills, while the older kids get, the more self-conscious they are about looking bad in front of their peers.

Research suggests that children are more likely to develop lifelong exercise habits when they have found activities they can be competent in, when those activities continue to be fun (and not a duty), and when they have ongoing support from parents, teachers, coaches, or peers. The best way parents can help is by setting an example, engaging in physical activities three to five times a week, until you all come to see exercise and physical activity as a normal part of your day or week.

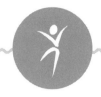

CHAPTER 13

Stay Healthy with Stretching

Stretching helps relieve stress, restlessness, or inattention. It's a good way to slowly warm up cold or unused muscles, particularly for kids or grown-ups with a history of inactivity. When done correctly, stretching will increase the range of motion in your joints, tendons, and muscles and allow you to do the exercises properly, reducing the risk of injuries, sprains, pulled muscles, or strained tendons.

You should spend about 10 minutes stretching before beginning your 30 minutes of exercise. With each stretch, push slowly against the tension without bouncing or rocking, breathing slowly and regularly through your nose as you do. If you feel significant discomfort, back off and don't push. Greater flexibility will come with repetition and patience, so don't try to do too much at once.

WHOLE BODY STRETCH. Stand with your feet shoulder-width apart. Raise both your arms overhead so that your hands are intertwined with palms together. Reach as high as you can and hold for 10 to 30 seconds, then relax.

ARM STRETCH. Stand with your feet shoulder-width apart and hold your arms straight out to the side with your palms facing up. Start moving your arms slowly in small circles and gradually make larger and larger circles. Come back to the starting position and reverse the direction of your arm swing. Do six to eight circles in one direction, then six to eight in the opposite direction.

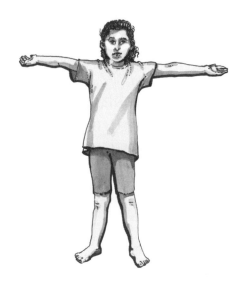

BACK STRETCH. Kneel on all fours. Raise first one arm and hold it out in front of you parallel to the floor, then return it to the floor. Do the same with your other arm. Next, raise one leg and hold it out straight behind you, parallel to the floor. Return to the all-fours position and then lift the other leg. Finally, raise one arm and one leg from opposite sides of your body and hold. Repeat with the other arm and leg. Do all movements slowly and hold for a few seconds.

LOWER BACK STRETCH. Lie on your back, with your knees bent and feet flat on the floor. Grasp one knee with both hands and pull it toward your chest until you feel the stretch. Hold for 10 seconds. Repeat with the other leg. Hold. Repeat with both knees at the same time, and hold for 10 seconds.

NECK STRETCH. While sitting or standing with your head in its normal upright position, slowly tilt it to the right until you feel tension on the left side of your neck. Hold that tension 10 to 30 seconds and then return your head to the upright position. Repeat to the left side, and then toward the front. Always return to the upright position before moving on, breathing slowly through your nose.

SIDE BEND. Stand with your feet shoulder-width apart and place your hands on your waist. Slowly bend to one side until you feel tension, keeping your neck straight. Hold 10 to 30 seconds and relax. Repeat on the other side.

HURDLER'S STRETCH. While seated, place one foot on the inside of the other leg just above your knee. Keep the other leg extended and straight. With your back straight, press forward toward the thigh of your extended leg. Use your hands for support. When you feel some tension in the back of your leg hold the stretch 15 to 20 seconds. Do not bounce while holding this stretch. Repeat twice with legs in each position.

GROIN STRETCH. Sit on a mat with your knees bent. Put the soles of your feet (or shoes) together and hold on to your ankles. Place your elbows inside your knees and slowly apply downward pressure until you feel tension. Hold 10 to 30 seconds and repeat.

Energize and Relax with Breathing

While you're stretching, focus on your breathing, particularly during the yoga-based stretches on pages 174–176. Take deep slow breaths, filling both the lower and upper regions of your lungs and neck; hold it for two or three seconds and then let it out slowly. Use your imagination. Imagine you're in the most peaceful place you know. Imagine how each inhalation brings oxygen to every cell of your body, and every exhalation removes stale air and impurities. Yoga is an ancient practice of focused breathing while holding poses that help stretch and bring energy to all parts of the body. In effect, it will provide additional mental health benefits and induce a relaxation response that can be helpful, particularly when we're feeling hungry.

CALF STRETCH. Face a wall, an arm's length away. Step back with one foot, keeping the other directly underneath you. Keep both feet pointing forward. Raise both arms and press your hands against the wall. Keeping both heels down, bend the front knee slightly. Then bend the knee of your back leg slightly until you feel that leg's calf stretch. Hold. Repeat with the other leg.

HAMSTRING STRETCH. Sit on the floor with your legs stretched out in a straddle position, feet spread wide. Stretch slowly to the right leg, bending at the waist while you attempt to touch your toes with both hands, reaching with your fingertips. Hold that position 10 to 15 seconds, breathing deeply in and out two to three times. Return to the center position, then turn to the left side and repeat. Stretch to each side five times.

HIP AND THIGH STRETCH. Stand sideways to a wall, an arm's length away. Place your hand on the wall for support. Lift the foot farthest from the wall. Hold the foot with your free hand so that your knee is pointing down. Gently pull your foot toward your buttocks, until you feel the stretch in the front of your leg. Hold for 10 seconds. Turn around and repeat the stretch on the other side. This can also be done lying on the floor on your side.

Yoga-Based Stretches

Yoga is based on a tradition of healthy body practices that dates back thousands of years. Many people have found great benefit from incorporating yoga into their daily activities. Be sure to focus on slow, steady breathing as you do these stretches.

COBRA STRETCH. Lie flat on your stomach on a pad or blanket, face down with your hands beside your chest. Keep your palms against the floor and your fingers pointing forward. Exhale and then, keeping flat on the floor, slide forward and lift your head and chest off the floor. Don't push with your hands, just let your spine lengthen and move like a snake. Keep your shoulders relaxed and your wrists down. To finish, bring your head and shoulders back to the floor, roll over and hug your knees to your chest.

SITTING TWIST. Sit up straight on a mat or folded blanket with your legs out in front of you. Sit evenly on both buttock bones, legs together, toes pointing up. Bring your right knee up close to your chest, keeping your other leg straight and flat to the floor. Hug your knee and straighten your spine. Exhale and turn your head and shoulders to the left so that your right arm goes around 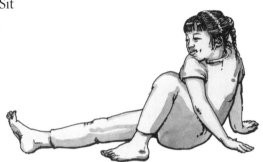 your bent leg. If you can, turn so that your left arm goes around the outside of your right leg. If you find this difficult, turn the other way, so that your right arm goes around the inside of your right leg. Bend your elbow and turn your arm around your bent leg until you can clasp your hands behind your back. Sit up as tall as you can, then unclasp your hands and reverse the pose.

CAT STRETCH. Kneel on all fours with the palms of your hands flat on the floor, your hands spaced shoulder-width apart. Your fingers should be pointing forward and your toes back. Keep your arms straight. As you exhale, hollow your back by pushing your belly toward the floor, keeping your arms straight and your shoulders relaxed. Inhale and when you next exhale, arch your back in the opposite direction. Return to your original position and repeat.

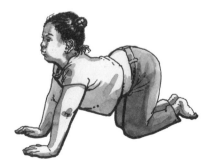 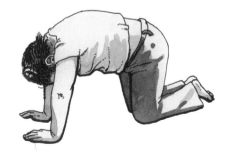

DOG STRETCH. Start on all fours with the palms of your hands and your knees on the floor, keeping your arms straight. Exhale. Tuck your toes under and lift up your hips and buttocks, slowly straightening your legs. Now stretch like a yawning dog until your arms and legs are straight with your weight back as far as you can make it on to your heels. Make sure that the right and left sides of your body stretch evenly and that you make a triangle with the floor. Bend your knees and sit gently down on your heels. Bend forward and relax.

WHAT PARENTS SHOULD KNOW

Children (and adults too) who are physically active can benefit in many ways from stretching. The most common reason for stretching is to increase flexibility, the ability to move joints through a full range of motion, in order to reduce the risk of injury. However, there are other benefits to stretching as well. By becoming more flexible through stretching, people can increase their power, sprint speed, and strength. For example, if a soccer player is able to move his or her leg farther back during the preparatory phase of a shot, more power can be applied. And runners can help optimize their personal speed by increasing their range of motion. Athletes with stretched muscles will also encounter less resistance from contraction and tension, which means that less energy is needed to complete a movement.

For a child or teen who is active in sports, failing to stretch can cause problems. Too little stretching can make your child more prone to muscle tears or strains and tendinitis, an overuse injury of the muscle tendon. For most children, there's little benefit to stretching before age 10, according to sports doctor Stephen Rice, MD, PhD, a spokesman for the American College of Sports Medicine. But starting earlier can get your children into the habit of stretching so that they'll be doing it when they need it. Accordingly, Mimi Johnson, MD, a member of an American Academy of Pediatrics sports medicine committee, recommends children begin stretching when they first join organized sports.

CHAPTER 14

Delicious Recipes

How many times have you looked at your watch, realized it's 6:30 in the evening, and you don't have anything at home to put on the table? It's a brave new world full of busy multitasking people, where parents and even kids share food preparation duties. Often the time needed to buy and prepare healthy food just isn't there, so we pick something up at McDonald's or we order a pizza.

Bad idea.

A return to the family table does not mean a return to the 1950s, or spending hours slaving in the kitchen. It means only planning a menu in advance, shopping once a week from a well-designed list, and occasionally precooking meals so that you don't find yourself scrambling to piece together a nourishing meal every night. It means taking control of your life. Cooking for your children is the best way to ensure they are eating well.

This chapter contains many healthy, low-fat, low-calorie recipes for you to try. The recipes were submitted by KidShape participants, who were asked to share a favorite food or dish, but to modify it to make it lower in fat or sugar. This means that the recipes have been tested by families and come recommended by kids who have lost weight eating them. At the end of each recipe, you will find useful information: the calories per serving, the grams of fat per serving, the percent of calories from fat, and a guide to how each food fits into your daily food guide pyramid.

You'll notice that many of the recipes call for readily available low-fat ingredients, such as low-fat cheese or nonfat yogurt. Some recipes also call for artificial sweeteners. Although it is not a good idea to use non-nutritive sweeteners excessively, one to two servings per day may be used. Those who do not wish to use artificial sweeteners may substitute an equivalent amount of sugar. And of course, remember to limit the portion size that you consume.

Appetizers

CHIPS AND DIP

1 teaspoon vanilla	½ cup nonfat plain yogurt
1 packet calorie-free sugar substitute	Dash of cinnamon
1 cup low-fat ricotta cheese	Red Delicious apples, thinly sliced

For the dip, mix together the vanilla, sweetener, ricotta cheese, yogurt, and cinnamon. Use the apple slices as chips. Serve at parties or at breakfast, chilled. *Makes 3 servings. Amount per serving:* Calories 232, Fat 7 g, % calories from fat 29.8%. *Food group servings per serving:* Fruit 2, Milk/yogurt 0.2, Protein 0.3, Fat/sweet 1.

TUNA PARTY DIP

1 (6-ounce) can tuna	¼ cup light cream cheese (Neufchatel)
⅓ cup nonfat plain yogurt	Salt and pepper, optional
Juice of 1 lemon, freshly squeezed	

Mix together in a bowl the tuna, yogurt, lemon juice, and cheese. Add salt and pepper if using. Arrange the spread over Swedish toast or low-fat whole-grain crackers. *Makes 8 servings. Amount per serving:* Calories 53, Fat 2.3 g, % calories from fat 39.1%. *Food group servings per serving:* Milk/yogurt 0.2, Protein 0.2, Fat/sweet 0.5.

EGGPLANT APPETIZER

2 cups water

2 cups chopped eggplant

2 cups chopped tomatoes

2 cups chopped onion

1 tablespoon extra-light olive oil

1 tablespoon crushed garlic

½ cup lemon juice

Put the water, eggplant, tomatoes, onion, and oil into a saucepan, and cook for 1 to 1½ hours. When the eggplant is done, add the garlic and lemon juice. Let the mixture chill. This dip can be eaten plain or with low-fat whole-grain crackers, meat, chicken, or potatoes. *Makes 8 servings.* *Amount per serving:* Calories 57, Fat 2 g, % calories from fat 31.5%. *Food group servings per serving:* Veg. 1, Fat/sweet 0.5.

HOT ARTICHOKE-CHILI DIP

1 can artichoke hearts, drained

4 ounces low-fat Cheddar cheese, grated

1 (4-ounce) can green chilies, chopped

Vegetables, crackers, or chips for serving

Process the artichoke hearts until smooth in a food processor Mix the cheese and chilies into the artichoke purée. Place in small, ovenproof crocks. To serve, heat through in the oven or microwave until the cheese melts. (Freeze any dip that you do not use.) Serve with vegetables, low-fat whole-grain crackers, or baked chips for dipping. *Makes 3 servings.* *Amount per serving:* Calories 183, Fat 7 g, % calories from fat 64%. *Food group servings per serving:* Protein 0.5, Fat/sweet 2.

SPINACH DIP

1 (6-ounce) can water chestnuts

1 (10-ounce) package frozen chopped
   spinach

1 envelope leek soup mix (do not mix
   according to directions)

1 cup nonfat sour cream

1 cup nonfat mayonnaise

Dash of Worcestershire sauce

Mix the water chestnuts, spinach, soup mix, sour cream, mayonnaise, and Worcestershire together and refrigerate. Serve with chips or Melba rounds. *Makes 8 servings.* Amount per serving: Calories 130.9, Fat 6.4 g, % calories from fat 44%. *Food group servings per serving:* Veg. 0.2, Protein 0.1, Fat/sweet 1.2.

Breads

TOFU BANANA BREAD

⅓ cup canola oil

1 cup regular tofu, mashed

1¼ cups sugar

2 eggs, slightly beaten

2 teaspoons vanilla

2 cups very ripe mashed bananas

2 tablespoons lemon juice

3½ cups all-purpose flour

2 teaspoons baking soda

1 teaspoon baking powder

1 teaspoon salt

1 cup chopped walnuts, optional

Preheat the oven to 350 degrees. Blend the oil and tofu in a food processor or blender until very smooth. Add the sugar, eggs, and vanilla and blend very well. Add the bananas and lemon juice, and process briefly. In a separate bowl combine the flour, baking soda, baking powder, and salt. Gently combine the liquid ingredients with the dry ingredients. Fold in the nuts, if using. Pour the batter into two, greased loaf pans. Bake for 50 to 60 minutes or until done, but not dry. *Makes 2 loaves/24 servings.* Amount per serving: Calories 182, Fat 6.6 g, % calories from fat 32.6%. *Food group servings per serving:* Grain 1, Protein 0.2, Fat/sweet 1.2.

CARROT BREAD

3 cups all-purpose flour

2 teaspoons soda

2 teaspoons cinnamon

2 teaspoons baking powder

1 cup sugar

1 teaspoon salt

4 cups egg beaters (equal to 4 eggs)

3 cups grated carrots

1½ cups applesauce

½ cup raisins

Preheat the oven to 350 degrees. Mix together in a large bowl the flour, soda, cinnamon, baking powder, sugar, and salt. Beat in the eggs, and add the carrots and applesauce. Mix well. Add the raisins and blend. Coat a loaf pan with nonfat cooking spray, and pour in the mixture. Bake 1 hour or until done, but not dry. Test with a straw or cake tester. *Makes l loaf/12 servings. Amount per serving:* Calories 306, Fat 3.2 g, % calories from fat 9.4%. *Food group servings per serving:* Grain 2, Veg. 0.5, Fat/sweet 1.

CORN BREAD

⅛ cup sugar

¼ cup canola oil

2 egg whites

½ cup all-purpose flour

¼ cup whole wheat flour

1½ teaspoons baking powder

Pinch of salt

¾ cup yellow cornmeal

½ cup nonfat milk

Preheat the oven to 400 degrees. Blend the sugar and oil in a medium bowl. Mix in the egg whites. Sift the flours with the baking powder and salt, and add the cornmeal. Blend the dry ingredients into the egg mixture alternately with milk. Spray a muffin tin with nonfat cooking spray, and dust with flour. Fill the muffin cups half full with the batter. Bake for 20 to 25 minutes. *Makes 8 muffins/ 8 servings. Amount per serving:* Calories 172, Fat 7 g, % calories from fat 36.6%. *Food group servings per serving:* Grain 1, Fat/sweet 1.4.

LEMON SQUASH MUFFINS

〜〜〜〜〜〜〜〜〜〜〜〜〜

2¼ cups all-purpose flour

1 teaspoon baking soda

1 teaspoon baking powder

¼ teaspoon salt

⅓ cup sugar

1 tablespoon canola oil

2 cups coarsely shredded summer squash (about ¾ pound), uncooked

1 tablespoon grated lemon rind

1 whole egg, lightly beaten

1 egg white, lightly beaten

1 (8-ounce) carton nonfat plain yogurt

Preheat the oven to 375 degrees. Combine the flour, baking soda, baking powder, salt, and sugar in a large bowl. Combine the oil with the squash, lemon rind, egg, egg white, and yogurt. Add the squash mixture to the dry ingredients, stirring just until moistened. Divide the batter evenly into a 12-cup muffin pan coated with nonfat cooking spray. Bake for 22 minutes. While the muffins cool slightly, prepare the Lemon Icing. Pierce the top of each muffin with a fork, and brush the muffins with the icing. Remove the muffins from the pan, and let them stand on a wire rack for 15 minutes. *Makes 12 muffins/12 servings.* *Amount per serving (includes icing):* Calories 145, Fat 2 g, % calories from fat 12.4%. *Food group servings per serving:* Grain 1, Fat/sweet 0.5.

LEMON ICING

3 tablespoons fresh lemon juice

2 tablespoons water

2 tablespoons sugar

Combine the lemon juice, water, and sugar in a small saucepan. Bring to a boil, and cook for 1 minute. Remove from the heat.

APPLE AND OAT BRAN MUFFINS

1¼ cups whole wheat flour

1 cup oat bran

⅓ cup packed brown sugar

2½ teaspoons baking powder

¼ teaspoon baking soda

¼ teaspoon salt

¼ teaspoon ground nutmeg

¼ teaspoon ground cinnamon

1 cup buttermilk

2 egg whites

2 tablespoons canola oil

¾ cup peeled and shredded apple

Preheat the oven to 375 degrees. In a medium bowl stir together the flour, oat bran, brown sugar, baking powder, baking soda, salt, nutmeg, and cinnamon. In a small bowl combine the buttermilk, egg whites, and oil. Add the buttermilk mixture to the dry ingredients, stirring just until moistened. Stir in the shredded apple. (You may store the batter, tightly covered, in the refrigerator for up to 5 days.) Coat a 12-cup muffin tin with nonfat cooking spray. Spoon about ¼ cup batter into each muffin cup. Bake for 18 to 20 minutes, or until a toothpick inserted near the center comes out clean. Cool slightly, and remove the muffins from the tin. *Makes 12 muffins/12 servings. Amount per serving:* Calories 124, Fat 3 g, % calories from fat 22%. *Food group servings per serving:* Grain 1, Protein 0.2, Fat/sweet 0.6.

Vegetables

FRIED RICE

2 cups boiled rice

1½ tablespoons canola oil

4 celery sticks, sliced

3 green onions, sliced

2 cups chopped broccoli

1 bell pepper, cut in small pieces

1½ cups chopped carrots

4 tablespoons soy sauce

When the rice is done, stir-fry it in the oil in a wok for 5 minutes along with the celery, onions, broccoli, pepper, and carrots. Season the mixture with the soy sauce. Serve with chicken breasts without skin to balance out the fat of the oil. *Makes 4 servings. Amount per serving:* Calories 190, Fat 6 g, % calories from fat 28.4%. *Food group servings per serving:* Grain 1.3, Fat/sweet 1.

GREEN BEANS AND RICE

1 tablespoon chopped garlic
2 cups cut green beans
Soy sauce

Black pepper
Boiled rice

Spray a saucepan with nonfat cooking spray, and sauté the chopped garlic. Add the green beans. Cook the beans, adding soy sauce and black pepper to taste. Stir and then cover the pan. When beans are crisp tender, serve hot with rice. *Makes 3 servings.* Amount per serving: Calories 118, Fat 0 g, % calories from fat 0%. *Food group servings per serving:* Grain 1, Veg. 1.

COLLARD GREENS AND POTATOES

2 bunches collard greens or a mixture
of collards and kale
3 medium gold potatoes
2 garlic cloves

1 medium onion
Salt
2 teaspoons canola oil
Pepper

Strip the collard leaves from the stems, and wash the greens. Scrub the potatoes, and dice coarsely. Finely dice the garlic cloves and onion. Bring 2 quarts of water to a boil in a large saucepan. Add the salt and greens, and simmer for 10 minutes. Scoop out the greens into a bowl. Add the potatoes to the water, and simmer until tender, 7 to 10 minutes. In a nonstick skillet, add the oil and heat. When the oil is hot, add the diced onion, and cook over medium-high heat for 5 minutes. Coarsely chop the cooked greens, and add them to the skillet along with the garlic. Add the pepper to taste and a little bit of the water from the potatoes, so that everything stays moist as it cooks. Add more water as needed. When the potatoes are tender, scoop them out of the pan, and add them to the greens. Season with the salt and add the pepper to taste. Serve with hot sauce or vinegar. *Makes 8 servings.* Amount per serving: Calories 86, Fat 1 g, % calories from fat 10.4%. *Food group servings per serving:* Grain 0.5, Veg. 1, Fat/sweet 0.2.

STIR-FRIED BROCCOLI

3 to 4 broccoli crowns

1 large piece ginger

2 tablespoons canola oil

½ teaspoon salt

1 tablespoon soy sauce

½ cup chicken broth

Wash the broccoli crowns, and cut them into florets. Peel and crush the ginger. Heat a wok or heavy skillet on high. Add the oil, and heat until smoking. Toss in the ginger, and press and turn it in the oil for a few seconds. Add the broccoli, and toss briskly to coat with the oil. When the broccoli is bright green, sprinkle with the salt, and drizzle the soy sauce down the side of the wok, tossing to combine with the broccoli. Pour in the chicken broth, and steam-cook, uncovered, for 2 minutes, stirring frequently. Serve immediately. *Makes 6 servings. Amount per serving:* Calories 56, Fat 5 g, % calories from fat 80%. *Food group servings per serving:* Veg. 1, Fat/sweet 1.

BAKED CARROT STICKS

2 pounds carrots

3 tablespoons margarine

1 teaspoon salt

Pepper

2 teaspoons sugar

⅓ cup orange juice

Preheat the oven to 400 degrees. Peel the carrots, and cut them into 2-inch sticks. Place the carrot sticks in a shallow casserole dish. Dot with the margarine, and sprinkle with the salt, pepper to taste, and sugar. Pour in the orange juice, cover with aluminum foil, and bake for 45 minutes, stirring occasionally. *Makes 8 servings. Amount per serving:* Calories 104, Fat 5 g, % calories from fat 43.2%. *Food group servings per serving:* Veg. 1.5, Fat/sweet 1.

Salads

CAESAR SALAD

¼ cup olive oil

1 clove garlic, crushed

Garlic powder

2 cups bread cubes

2 heads romaine lettuce

1 head Boston lettuce

¾ cup freshly grated Parmesan cheese

½ teaspoon salt

¼ teaspoon dry mustard

¼ teaspoon freshly ground pepper

⅓ cup lemon juice

2 eggs

Dash of Worcestershire sauce

Pour the oil into a jar, and add the garlic. Cover and let stand for at least 1 hour. Preheat the oven to 350 degrees. Sprinkle the garlic powder to taste on the bread cubes, and bake for 5 minutes. Tear the romaine and Boston lettuce into a large salad bowl. Combine the cheese, salt, mustard, and pepper. Boil water in a small saucepan. Place the eggs in their shells into the boiling water for 1 minute. Remove the eggs and place them briefly in cold water to cool. Break the eggs into a medium bowl. Beat the lemon juice gradually into the eggs, and then add the Worcestershire sauce, the garlic/oil, and the cheese mixture. Pour one-third of the dressing over the salad, and toss gently. Add the croutons during the last tossing. Serve immediately. *Makes 12 servings.* Amount per serving: Calories 103, Fat 7.6 g, % calories from fat 66.4%. *Food group servings per serving:* Grain 0.2, Veg. 2, Protein 0.2, Fat/sweet 1.

JAPANESE-STYLE CUCUMBERS

2 large cucumbers

4 green onions

⅓ cup sweetened rice wine vinegar

Peel and thinly slice the cucumbers. Then thinly slice the white part of the onions and two or three inches of the green part. Mix the cucumbers and onions together in a medium-size bowl with the vinegar, and chill for 1 to 2 hours. *Makes 4 servings.* Amount per serving: Calories 29, Fat 0 g, % calories from fat 0%. *Food group servings per serving:* Veg. 2.

NANA SHEILA'S FRUIT SALAD

3 cups shredded lettuce

1 pint strawberries, halved

1 large banana, sliced

1 honeydew melon, cubed

1 (20-ounce) can pineapple chunks, juice drained.

1 (8-ounce) carton nonfat vanilla yogurt

½ cup shredded Gruyere cheese

In a large bowl put half the lettuce. Layer the strawberries, banana, melon, and pineapple on top of the lettuce bed. Top with the remaining lettuce, and spread the yogurt over the top. Sprinkle with the cheese. Cover and chill 2 to 3 hours. Toss gently to serve. *Makes 12 servings.* Amount per serving: Calories 145.4, Fat 1.7 g, % calories from fat 10.5%. *Food group servings per serving:* Fruit 2, Milk/yogurt 0.2, Protein 0.2, Fat/sweet 1.

GREEN AND ORANGE SALAD

2 navel oranges, peeled

1 large head Boston lettuce

2 small green onions, sliced

4 slices avocado

Divide the oranges into sections, reserving four sections for the dressing. Cut the sections into bite-size pieces. Tear the lettuce into bite-size pieces. Arrange the lettuce at the bottom of a salad bowl, and place the other orange sections, green onions, and avocado slices on top. Prepare the Orange-Honey Dressing. Pour the dressing over the salad, and toss lightly to mix. *Makes 4 servings.* Amount per serving (includes dressing): Calories 80, Fat 6 g, % calories from fat 67.5%. *Food group servings per serving:* Veg. 2, Fruit 0.5, Fat/sweet 1.

ORANGE HONEY DRESSING

1 tablespoon canola oil

1 teaspoon honey

2 tablespoons cider vinegar

4 orange sections

Blend the oil, honey, vinegar, and orange sections together in a bowl.

HOMETOWN SALAD

1 clove garlic, cut

4 hard-cooked eggs

1 tablespoon canola oil

4 tablespoons cider vinegar

Salt and pepper

1 head butter lettuce

Rub a salad bowl with the cut clove of garlic. Peel and slice the eggs, separating the yolks from the whites. Put the yolks into the salad bowl, and add the oil and vinegar. Mix until the egg yolks are smooth and completely blended with the oil and vinegar. Add salt and pepper to taste. Break up the lettuce leaves, add them to the salad bowl along with the sliced egg whites, and toss lightly. *Makes 4 servings.* Amount per serving: Calories 128, Fat 10 g, % calories from fat 70.3%. *Food group servings per serving:* Veg. 1, Protein 1, Fat/sweet 1.

JUNE'S SALAD

1 (16-ounce) package chow mein noodles

1 head cabbage

4 green onions

2 tablespoons sesame seeds

Prepare and refrigerate the Asian Dressing. For the salad, crumble the noodles into small pieces. Chop the cabbage, and thinly slice the green onions. In a toaster oven, toast the sesame seeds until lightly browned. Combine the noodles with the sesame seeds. Place the cabbage in a salad bowl, and sprinkle the onion slices on top. Sprinkle the dried noodle mixture over the cabbage and onions, and pour the dressing over all. Toss well and serve immediately. *Makes 8 servings.* Amount per serving (includes dressing): Calories 235, Fat 15.2 g, % calories from fat 58%. *Food group servings per serving:* Grain 1, Veg. 1, Protein 0.2, Fat/sweet 2.

ASIAN DRESSING

1 tablespoon canola oil

2 tablespoons vinegar

1 tablespoon soy sauce

¼ teaspoon powdered ginger

2 tablespoons sugar

Salt and pepper

For the dressing, combine the oil, vinegar, soy sauce, ginger, and sugar, and add the salt and pepper to taste. Mix well.

Entrées

LETTUCE BUNDLES WITH HOT-AND-SWEET MEAT FILLING

2 teaspoons sesame oil

½ pound lean ground beef

4 scallions, trimmed and finely sliced
    on the diagonal, divided

½ cup rice wine or dry sherry

4 tablespoons kochujang or Chinese
    chili paste with garlic

4 cloves garlic, finely chopped

2 tablespoons peeled and finely
    chopped gingerroot

2 tablespoons sugar

2 heads Boston lettuce, leaves sepa-
    rated and washed

2 cups steamed white rice

Heat the oil in a small, nonstick sauté pan. Add the ground beef, and cook 2 to 3 minutes. Drain the fat from the meat. Add half the scallions, the wine or sherry, kochujang or Chinese chili paste, garlic, ginger, and sugar to the pan. Cook over very low heat for 7 to 10 minutes. Spoon the meat mixture into a small bowl. (The filling can be made up to 2 days in advance if refrigerated and covered. Serve warm.) Arrange the lettuce leaves on a platter, sprinkle the remaining scallions over the meat, and serve along with the rice. Guests can make up their own bundles. *Makes 6 servings.* Amount per serving: Calories 412, Fat 10.7 g, % calories from fat 23.6%. *Food group servings per serving:* Grain 2, Veg. 1, Protein 1, Fat/sweet 2.

EMILY'S BREAD-SLICE BURRITOS

1 tablespoon fat-free, refried beans

1 tablespoon browned, lean ground
    beef

½ to 1 slice low-fat mozzarella cheese

1 slice light honey-bran or wheat bread,
    crust trimmed

Put the beans, beef, and cheese in a microwave-safe bowl. Heat in the microwave on high for 30 seconds or until the cheese is melted. Spread the mixture on top of the bread. *Makes 1 serving.* Amount per serving: Calories 247, Fat 10.8 g, % calories from fat 39.3%. *Food group servings per serving:* Grain 1, Protein 1, Fat/sweet 2.

BLACK BEAN ENCHILADA PIE

~~~~~~~~~~~~~~~~~~~~~~~

1 tablespoon canola oil

1 onion, peeled and chopped

1 jalapeño pepper, seeded and cut into slivers

2 garlic cloves, peeled and finely minced

½ teaspoon ground cumin

Salt and pepper

2 (16-ounce) cans black beans, rinsed and drained

1 (15-ounce) can tomato sauce

2 (14-ounce) cans Mexican-style corn, drained

4 green onions, sliced, plus additional for topping

4 large low-fat flour tortillas, made without lard

2½ cups grated low-fat Monterey Jack cheese

Low-fat sour cream and salsa for garnishes

Preheat the oven to 400 degrees. Heat the oil in a skillet over medium heat. Sauté the onion, jalapeño, and garlic for 1 to 2 minutes. Add the cumin and the salt and pepper to taste, and cook until the onion is soft, 5 to 7 minutes. Add the beans and tomato sauce, and bring to a boil. Cook until the liquid is almost gone, about 8 to 10 minutes. Stir in the corn and the 4 green onions, and remove from the heat. Check the mixture, and season to taste with additional salt and pepper. In a pie dish, place 1 tortilla on the bottom, top with one-fourth of the bean mixture and ½ cup of the cheese. Repeat three times, topping with the remaining ½ cup cheese. Bake until hot and the cheese is melted, about 20 to 25 minutes. Sprinkle with the additional chopped green onions, cut into wedges, and serve with garnishes, including sour cream and salsa. *Makes 8 servings.* Amount per serving: Calories 418, Fat 15 g, % calories from fat 32.2%. *Food group servings per serving:* Grain 2, Protein 1, Fat/sweet 3.

LONDON BROIL

~~~~~~~~~~~~~~~~~~~~~~~

2½ pounds London broil steak

½ teaspoon garlic salt

½ teaspoon pepper

Salt

Preheat the oven to 350 degrees. Season the meat to taste, and bake for 1 hour. *Makes 8 servings.* Amount per serving: Calories 279, Fat 11 g, % calories from fat 35.5%. *Food group servings per serving:* Protein 1.5, Fat/sweet 2.

LEMON CHICKEN

1 pound skinless chicken pieces

3 tablespoons low-sodium soy sauce

2 teaspoons Mrs. Dash seasoning

Juice of 1½ lemons

1 tablespoon margarine

Cooked rice for serving

Wash and rinse the chicken pieces, and place them in a shallow baking dish. Combine the soy sauce, Mrs. Dash, and lemon juice. Pour over the chicken pieces, and let stand for 1 hour in the refrigerator. When ready to cook, preheat the oven to 350 degrees, and remove the chicken from the refrigerator. Pat the margarine on top of the chicken. Bake for 1 hour, or until the juices run clear when tested with a fork. Serve on a bed of steamed rice. *Makes 6 servings.* Amount per serving: Calories 420, Fat 11.2 g, % calories from fat 24.1%. *Food group servings per serving:* Grain 2, Protein 1, Fat/sweet 2.

SPICY JAMAICAN JERK CHICKEN

1 tablespoon Tabasco sauce

3 tablespoons Worcestershire sauce

1 tablespoon A-1 sauce

1 cup Jamaican jerk sauce

½ cup parsley flakes

½ cup minced onion

1 whole chicken, cut into pieces and
   skin removed

For the marinade, combine the Tabasco, Worcestershire, A-1, and jerk sauces with the parsley and onion. Marinate the chicken in the refrigerator for 8 to 10 hours or overnight. Remove the chicken from the marinade, and grill or bake in a 350-degree oven until the juices run clear when tested with a fork. *Makes 8 servings.* Amount per serving: Calories 146, Fat 4.9 g, % calories from fat 30.2%. *Food group servings per serving:* Grain 0.2, Protein 1, Fat/sweet 1.

CHICKEN AND NOODLES

2 skinless, boneless chicken breasts,
   cut into pieces
1 small onion, quartered
1 rib celery, cut in pieces
1 small green pepper, seeded and
   quartered
Salt and pepper

1 chicken bouillon cube, optional
1 (8-ounce) package egg noodles,
   cooked according to package
   directions
1 (10¾-ounce) can low-fat cream of
   celery, chicken, or mushroom soup
1 cup grated low-fat Cheddar cheese

Boil the chicken in water to cover, with the onion, celery, green pepper, and salt and pepper to taste. Add the chicken bouillon cube, if using. When the chicken is done, drain all but 1 cup of broth, and add the noodles and can of soup. Preheat the oven to 350 degrees. Pour the mixture into a casserole dish, and top with the cheese. Bake for 20 to 25 minutes. **Makes 8 servings.** Amount per serving: Calories 213, Fat 4.9 g, % calories from fat 20.7%. Food group servings per serving: Grain 1, Veg. 0.5, Protein 0.7, Fat/sweet 1.

EMILY'S BAKED BREADED CHICKEN

2 boneless, skinless chicken breasts
2 cups nonfat milk
1 cup plain breadcrumbs

½ teaspoon salt
2 tablespoons margarine

Preheat the oven to 400 degrees. Trim all the fat off the chicken, and cut the breasts into 1- to 2-ounce pieces. Place the chicken between two pieces of waxed paper, and pound to about ¼ inch thick. Place the pieces in the milk, one at a time, to coat. Then dredge the chicken in the breadcrumbs, one at a time, turning and coating well. Place the chicken pieces into a baking pan that has been coated with nonfat cooking spray. Lightly sprinkle the chicken with the salt, and dot each piece with a small amount of margarine. Bake for 25 minutes. **Makes 4 servings.** Amount per serving: Calories 255, Fat 9.1 g, % calories from fat 32.1%. Food group servings per serving: Grain 0.5, Protein 1, Fat/sweet 1.

CHICKEN PIZZA

5 cloves garlic, finely chopped

1 tomato, finely chopped

1 cup cooked chicken, chopped

1 cup chopped cilantro

½ onion, finely chopped

1 prepared (16-inch) pizza dough

Preheat the oven to 400 degrees. Sprinkle the garlic, tomato, chicken, cilantro, and onion over the pizza dough, and bake for 10 to 15 minutes. *Makes 4 servings.* Amount per serving: Calories 395, Fat 9.1 g, % calories from fat 32.2%. Food group servings per serving: Grain 2.5, Veg. 0.5, Protein 1, Fat/sweet 1.6.

CHICKEN TOSTADAS

2 whole chicken breasts, skin and fat
    removed

2 cloves garlic

1 onion, chopped

½ teaspoon ground cumin

1 teaspoon cilantro leaves

4 cups water

4 corn tortillas

1 can nonfat refried beans

1 head lettuce, shredded

3 tomatoes, chopped

1 cup low-fat Cheddar cheese, shredded

Combine the chicken, garlic, onion, cumin, cilantro, and water, and boil for 25 minutes. Remove the chicken breasts, and allow to cool. Preheat the oven to 350 degrees. Shred the chicken. Heat the tortillas in the oven for 8 minutes. Remove from the oven, and spread each tortilla with 1 tablespoon refried beans. Top with lettuce, tomato, cheese, and ½ cup shredded chicken. This is good served with saffron rice, black beans, and sliced pineapple. *Makes 4 servings.* Amount per serving: Calories 480, Fat 16 g, % calories from fat 30%. Food group servings per serving: Grain 3, Veg. 2, Protein 1.2, Fat/sweet 3.

SALMON PATTIES

1 (1-pound) can salmon
2 eggs

½ cup breadcrumbs

Preheat the oven to 350 degrees. Remove the bones from the salmon, and mash with the eggs and breadcrumbs. Form into 6 patties, and bake until heated through. *Makes 6 servings.* Amount per serving: Calories 126.6, Fat 6 g, % calories from fat 42.6%. *Food group servings per serving:* Grain 0.1, Protein 1, Fat/sweet 1.

TUNA CASSEROLE

8 ounces noodles or pasta
1 (10¾-ounce) can low-fat cream of
    mushroom soup
½ to ¾ cup nonfat milk
1 (6-ounce) can tuna fish in water,
    drained

½ cup frozen peas
¼ to ½ teaspoon dried dill weed
¼ teaspoon garlic powder
⅛ teaspoon black or white pepper
½ to ¾ cup shredded low-fat
    mozzarella cheese

Cook the noodles or pasta according to package directions. Set aside to drain. Preheat the oven to 350 degrees. In a large bowl mix the soup and milk. Add the tuna, peas, dill, garlic powder, and pepper. Combine with the drained noodles. Pour the mixture into a 2-quart casserole dish, and top with the cheese. Cook in the oven until hot and bubbly on the edges, about 30 minutes. You can use turkey or chicken breasts (⅔ cup) instead of tuna. *Makes 6 servings.* Amount per serving: Calories 233, Fat 5.2 g, % calories from fat 20%. *Food group servings per serving:* Grain 1, Protein 0.5, Fat/sweet 1.

EGGPLANT PARMESAN

4 egg whites plus 2 whole eggs, slightly beaten	1 medium-size eggplant, cut in ¼-inch-thick rounds
¼ cup nonfat milk	1½ cups tomato sauce
½ cup whole wheat flour	¼ teaspoon oregano
1 plus ½ teaspoon salt	Dash of black pepper
2½ cups crushed whole wheat crackers	½ cup grated Parmesan cheese, divided
	1 cup grated low-fat mozzarella cheese

Mix the eggs with the milk. Prepare three bowls for dipping the eggplant slices: the first containing the whole wheat flour and 1 teaspoon salt, the second containing the eggs and milk, and the third containing the cracker crumbs. Preheat the oven to 350 degrees. Dredge the eggplant slices first in the flour, then in the eggs, and then in the crushed cracker crumbs, coating the eggplant completely. Layer the slices in a 9 x 13-inch glass dish. Slices may overlap, but they should not cover each other completely. Mix the tomato sauce with the remaining ½ teaspoon salt, oregano, and black pepper. Sprinkle each eggplant layer with the tomato sauce and half the Parmesan cheese. Cover tightly, and bake for 30 to 45 minutes, or until a fork pierces the middle slices easily. Top with the mozzarella cheese and the remaining Parmesan cheese. Return the dish to the oven, and cook, uncovered, just until the cheese melts. *Makes 6 servings.* Amount per serving: Calories 345, Fat 12.9 g, % calories from fat 33.6%. *Food group servings per serving:* Grain 1.8, Veg. 1, Protein 0.6, Fat/sweet 2.5.

ENGLISH MUFFIN PIZZAS

1 whole wheat English muffin, split	2 slices low-fat mozzarella cheese, broken in pieces
½ cup pizza sauce, divided	

Spread each muffin half with ¼ cup pizza sauce. Top each with half the cheese, and toast for 3 to 5 minutes in a toaster oven. *Makes 2 servings.* Amount per serving: Calories 190, Fat 8 g, % calories from fat 37.8%. *Food group servings per serving:* Grain 1, Protein 0.5, Fat/sweet 1.

QUICK VEGETABLE PIZZA
~~~~~~~~~~~~~~~~

1 prepared (16-inch) pizza dough	½ cup sliced plum tomatoes
¾ cup tomato sauce	½ cup sliced zucchini rounds
¾ cup shredded low-fat mozzarella cheese	½ cup sliced onion
	½ cup sliced mushrooms
¾ cup grated Parmesan cheese	½ cup sliced green pepper

Preheat the oven to 450 degrees. Brush or spread the pizza dough with the tomato sauce. Sprinkle with half the mozzarella and half the Parmesan cheese. Arrange the tomato slices over the pizza crust, and top with the zucchini, onion, mushrooms, and green pepper. Sprinkle on the remaining half of the cheeses. Place the pizza on a cookie sheet or pizza stone, and bake for 10 to 12 minutes. *Makes 4 servings. Amount per serving:* Calories 507, Fat 16 g, % calories from fat 28.4%. *Food group servings per serving:* Grain 2.6, Veg. 1, Protein 1, Fat/sweet 3.

STUFFED SHELLS
~~~~~~~~~~~~~~~~

¾ pound large pasta shells	1 jar or large can of spaghetti sauce
12 ounces nonfat cottage cheese	Fresh garlic
10 ounces low-fat ricotta cheese	Black pepper
2 ounces low-fat garlic Jack cheese, finely chopped or grated	Assorted spices

Boil the shells in a large pan of water for 4 to 5 minutes, or until slightly pliable, but very undercooked. Rinse with cold water. Preheat the oven to 300 degrees. Mix together the cottage cheese, ricotta cheese, and Jack cheese thoroughly. Fill each of the shells with approximately 1 heaping tablespoon of the cheese stuffing mix. Arrange the shells in a nonstick baking pan. Season the spaghetti sauce with the garlic, pepper, and spices to taste. Pour the sauce over the shells. Cover the pan tightly with aluminum foil, and bake 30 minutes. To extend the stuffing, add oil-free sautéed mushrooms, spinach, or other vegetables. *Makes 6 servings. Amount per serving:* Calories 352, Fat 15.8 g, % calories from fat 40.4%. *Food group servings per serving:* Grain 1.4, Protein 0.7, Fat/sweet 1.

NOODLE KUGEL

1 pound medium-size noodles (not egg
   noodles)

8 egg whites

1 quart buttermilk

½ stick butter or margarine, melted

¼ cup sugar

Cook the noodles according to package directions. Preheat the oven to 350 degrees. Mix in a large bowl the egg whites, buttermilk, butter, and sugar. Add the cooked noodles. Grease a 9 x 13-inch pan, pour in the noodle mix, and place in the oven. Prepare the Cornflake Topping. After the pudding has baked for 45 minutes, sprinkle the topping on it. Then bake for an additional 30 minutes. *Makes 8 servings. Amount per serving (includes topping):* Calories 337, Fat 4.7 g, % calories from fat 34.1%. *Food group servings per serving:* Grain 2, Protein 0.5, Fat/sweet 3.

CORNFLAKE TOPPING

1 tablespoon butter or margarine

¼ cup brown sugar

1 cup crushed cornflakes

Melt the butter, add the brown sugar and cornflakes, and mix.

Desserts

RACHEL LENDER'S STRAWBERRY SPREAD

10 fresh strawberries

1 banana

1 cup nonfat cottage cheese

1 teaspoon vanilla extract

Dash of cinnamon

Mash the strawberries and banana together, and combine with the cottage cheese and vanilla in a blender. Process for approximately 2 minutes until smooth. Sprinkle on the cinnamon. Spread the fruit mixture on toast or crackers. *Makes 32 (1-tablespoon) servings. Amount per serving:* Calories 14, Fat 1 g, % calories from fat 45.9%. *Food group servings per serving:* Fruit 0.2, Fat/sweet 1.

CARROT CAKE
~~~~~~~~~~

2 cups all-purpose flour (or half whole
   wheat, half all-purpose)

1 cup sugar

1 teaspoon salt

2 teaspoons cinnamon

1 cup applesauce

1 cup canola oil

2 whole eggs and 4 egg whites

3 cups grated carrots (about 1 pound)

Preheat the oven to 350 degrees. In a large bowl, sift together the flour, sugar, salt, and cinnamon. In a medium bowl, mix the applesauce and oil together for 5 minutes, and then add to the flour mixture. Beat in the eggs, one at a time, and fold in the carrots. Pour the cake batter into three layer pans, and bake 30 to 35 minutes. Cool. Prepare Cream Cheese Icing, and spread on the cake layers. *Makes 12 servings. Amount per serving (includes icing): Calories 403, Fat 25.2 g, % calories from fat 56.3%. Food group servings per serving: Grain 1.6, Veg. 0.5, Protein 0.2, Fat/sweet 5.*

CREAM CHEESE ICING

8 ounces light cream cheese
   (Neufchatel)

4 teaspoons vanilla extract

4 teaspoons calorie-free sugar
   substitute

1 cup fat-free tub margarine

Cream together the cheese, vanilla, sweetener, and margarine.

YOGURT BROWNIES
~~~~~~~~~~

1 box brownie mix

½ cup nonfat plain yogurt

Prepare the brownie mix according to the directions on the box, but substitute the yogurt for the cooking oil and eggs. Bake in a 9 x 13-inch pan. *Makes 24 brownies/24 servings. Amount per serving: Calories 124, Fat 1 g, % calories from fat 7.3%. Food group servings per serving: Grain 1.2, Protein 0.2.*

CHOCOLATE CAKE

1½ cups cake flour

½ cup whole wheat flour

1 cup packed brown sugar

2 teaspoons baking soda

2 teaspoons baking powder

2 cups water

⅔ cup unsweetened cocoa powder

½ cup margarine

¼ cup nonfat plain yogurt

½ cup banana purée

Preheat the oven to 375 degrees. Sift the flours, sugar, baking soda, and baking powder into a large bowl. Combine the water, cocoa, and margarine in a saucepan. Heat and stir until the margarine is melted and the cocoa is dissolved. Combine the cocoa mixture with the flour mixture. Mix the yogurt and banana purée with a wire whisk in a separate bowl until creamy. Add the yogurt/banana to the batter, and mix gently until blended. Pour into a 9 x 13-inch cake pan sprayed with nonfat cooking spray. Bake 40 to 45 minutes, or until a toothpick inserted in the center of the cake comes out clean. ***Makes 15 servings.*** *Amount per serving:* Calories 185, Fat 6.9 g, % calories from fat 33.6%. *Food group servings per serving:* Grain 1.2, Protein 0.1, Fat/sweet 1.4.

SWEET POTATO PUFF

3 cups fresh sweet potatoes, cooked
    and peeled

4 egg whites

2 plus 3 tablespoons all-purpose flour

¼ cup granulated sugar

1 teaspoon vanilla

½ cup brown sugar

2 tablespoons margarine

½ cup chopped pecans

Preheat the oven to 350 degrees. Coat a 1½-quart casserole dish with nonfat cooking spray. Using a food processor or mixer, blend the sweet potatoes with the egg whites, 2 tablespoons flour, the granulated sugar, and vanilla until smooth. Pour into the casserole. Crumble the remaining 3 tablespoons flour, brown sugar, and margarine in a small bowl, and stir in the pecans. Sprinkle the pecan mixture over the sweet potato mixture. Bake for 30 minutes until golden brown. ***Makes 6 servings.*** *Amount per serving:* Calories 231, Fat 10.2 g, % calories from fat 39.7%. *Food group servings per serving:* Grain 1.3, Protein 0.2, Fat/sweet 2.

OATMEAL DATE COOKIES

2 cups oatmeal or rolled oats	2 teaspoons vanilla
⅔ cup pitted dates	½ cup canola oil
2 tablespoons brown sugar	½ teaspoon salt
4 egg whites (or 4 tablespoons pow- dered egg white and ½ cup water)	½ cup chopped walnuts

Preheat the oven to 350 degrees. In a blender, combine the oats, dates, and brown sugar until the consistency of flour. Combine the egg whites, vanilla, oil, and salt in a bowl, and mix well. Add the walnuts, and then add the oatmeal and date mixture. Coat a cookie sheet with nonfat cooking spray. Drop the mixture by tablespoonfuls onto the cookie sheet to make 20 cookies. Flatten the dollops of dough with a fork dipped in flour. Bake for 10 to 12 minutes. *Makes 20 cookies/ 20 servings. Amount per serving:* Calories 112, Fat 8.2 g, % calories from fat 66%. *Food group servings per serving:* Grain 0.4, Fat/sweet 2.

CHOCOLATE CHIP COOKIES

½ stick margarine	1 teaspoon baking soda
⅔ cup granulated sugar	2¼ cups all-purpose flour
⅔ cup brown sugar	2 egg whites
1 teaspoon vanilla extract	1 (12-ounce) bag chocolate chips
1 teaspoon salt	

Preheat the oven to 375 degrees. Mix the margarine, sugars, and vanilla in a mixer until smooth. In a separate bowl, combine the salt, baking soda, and flour. Add the egg whites to the sugar mixture, and beat until smooth. Add the flour mixture and beat. Add the chocolate chips. Grease a cookie sheet with nonfat cooking spray and drop 1 heaping teaspoon of dough for each cookie. Bake 9 to 10 minutes. *Makes 60 cookies/60 servings. Amount per serving:* Calories 69, Fat 2.5 g, % calories from fat 32.5%. *Food group servings per serving:* Grain 2, Fat/sweet 0.5.

EASY FRUIT SOUFFLÉ

1 cup nonfat milk

¼ cup cornstarch

1½ cups fresh fruit

⅓ cup sugar (or Splenda)

1 teaspoon vanilla

1 cup egg substitute

2 egg whites

In a small saucepan gradually blend the milk and cornstarch. Cook over medium heat, stirring constantly, until the mixture thickens and begins to boil. Remove from the heat, and stir in the fruit, sugar, and vanilla. In a medium bowl, with an electric mixer on high, beat the egg substitute until foamy, about 3 minutes, and then fold the egg substitute into the fruit mixture. Beat the egg whites, and fold into the fruit. Preheat the oven to 375 degrees. Spoon the mixture into a 1-quart soufflé or casserole dish that has been coated with nonfat cooking spray. Bake 45 to 50 minutes or until set. Serve immediately. ***Makes 6 servings.*** *Amount per serving:* Calories 137, Fat 2.6 g, % calories from fat 17.1%. *Food group servings per serving:* Fruit 1, Protein 0.3, Fat/sweet 0.5.

PUMPKIN CUPCAKES

1¾ cups all-purpose flour, sifted

1¼ cups sugar

1 teaspoon baking soda

¾ teaspoon salt

½ teaspoon ginger

½ teaspoon cinnamon

½ teaspoon allspice

2 teaspoons nutmeg

1 cup canned pumpkin

½ cup canola oil

⅓ cup water

2 eggs

Preheat the oven to 350 degrees. In a medium bowl, combine the flour, sugar, baking soda, salt, ginger, cinnamon, allspice, and nutmeg. In a large bowl, combine the pumpkin, oil, water, and eggs, and mix well. Add the flour mixture to the pumpkin mixture, and mix. Pour the batter into greased muffin cups, and bake 20 to 25 minutes. Place on a cake rack to cool. ***Makes 12 cupcakes/12 servings.*** *Amount per serving:* Calories 249, Fat 10.3 g, % calories from fat 37.3%. *Food group servings per serving:* Grain 1.5, Protein 0.1, Fat/sweet 2.

DESSERT NACHOS WITH FRUIT SALSA AND YOGURT TOPPING

2 large kiwi fruits, peeled and diced

2 cups strawberries, hulled and rinsed

1 (11-ounce) can mandarin oranges, drained

2 tablespoons ground cinnamon

10 (8-inch) flour tortillas

1 cup plain nonfat yogurt mixed with 1 packet calorie-free sugar substitute

½ cup orange juice

3 tablespoons honey

Combine the kiwi, strawberries, and oranges in a separate bowl for a fruit salsa. Preheat the oven to 500 degrees. Put the cinnamon in a shallow bowl. Working with one tortilla at a time, brush both sides lightly with water, and then cut into six equal wedges. Dip one side of each wedge in the cinnamon. Arrange in a single layer, cinnamon side up, on tinfoil-lined baking sheets coated with nonfat cooking spray. Bake until crisp and golden, 4 to 5 minutes. In a small bowl, combine the yogurt, orange juice, and honey to make the yogurt topping. Mound the tortilla chips on a large platter, and serve with the fruit salsa and the yogurt topping on the side. *Makes 10 servings.* Amount per serving: Calories 160, Fat 1.9 g, % calories from fat 10.7%. *Food group servings per serving:* Grain 1.3, Fruit 0.5, Milk/yogurt 0.1, Fat/sweet 0.2.

Drinks

BREAKFAST SMOOTHIE

3 to 6 ice cubes

1 banana

½ cup nonfat plain yogurt

½ cup pineapple or orange juice

In a blender, combine the ice cubes, banana, yogurt, and juice. Blend until smooth. For a thinner shake, use six ice cubes. *Makes 1 serving.* Amount per serving: Calories 231, Fat 0.8 g, % calories from fat 3.1%. *Food group servings per serving:* Fruit 3, Milk/yogurt 0.5, Fat/sweet 0.2.

STRAWBERRY FRUIT SMOOTHIE

2 cups (1-pint basket) strawberries

1 cup nonfat vanilla yogurt

1 cup crushed ice

½ cup orange juice

Calorie-free sugar substitute

In a blender, mix together the strawberries, yogurt, ice, juice, and the sweetener to taste. Process for 30 seconds. *Makes 4 servings.* Amount per serving: Calories 92, Fat 0.5 g, % calories from fat 4.9%. *Food group servings per serving:* Fruit 1.5, Milk/yogurt 0.3, Protein 0.1, Fat/sweet 0.1.

PEACH SMOOTHIE

3 peaches, peeled and pitted

1 cup nonfat vanilla yogurt

½ cup orange juice

1 cup crushed ice

Calorie-free sugar substitute

In a blender, mix together the peaches, yogurt, orange juice, ice, and the sweetener to taste. Process for 30 seconds. *Makes 4 servings.* Amount per serving: Calories 91, Fat 0.2 g, % calories from fat 1.9%. *Food group servings per serving:* Fruit 1, Milk/yogurt 0.3, Fat/sweet 0.1.

BERRY GOOD STRAWBERRY SMOOTHIE

2 cups (1-pint basket) strawberries

1 cup nonfat milk

1 cup nonfat plain yogurt

1 packet calorie-free sugar substitute

Wash and cut off the tops of the strawberries, if using fresh strawberries. Put the strawberries into a blender with the milk, yogurt, and sweetener, and blend. *Makes 4 servings.* Amount per serving: Calories 78, Fat 0.5 g, % calories from fat 5.7%. *Food group servings per serving:* Fruit 1, Milk/yogurt 0.3, Fat/sweet 0.1.

BANANA-STRAWBERRY SMOOTHIE

~~~~~~~~~~~~~~~~~~~~~~~~~~~~~~~~~~~~~

4 to 5 strawberries   ¼ to ½ cup orange juice

1 banana   12 ice cubes

In a blender, combine the strawberries, banana, orange juice, and ice cubes. Process until thick. *Makes 2 servings. Amount per serving:* Calories 86, Fat 0.5 g, % calories from fat 4.5%. *Food group servings per serving:* Fruit 1, Fat/sweet 1.

HEALTHY MILK SHAKE

~~~~~~~~~~~~~~~~~~~~~~~~~~~~~~~~~~~~~

2 packets calorie-free sugar substitute   1 cup nonfat vanilla or other flavor

2 cups nonfat milk   yogurt

In a blender, combine the sweetener, milk, and yogurt. Process for 1 minute. *Makes 3 servings. Amount per serving:* Calories 126, Fat 0.4 g, % calories from fat 2.8%. *Food group servings per serving:* Milk/yogurt 0.5, Fat/sweet 0.1.

LIMEADE COOLER

~~~~~~~~~~~~~~~~~~~~~~~~~~~~~~~~~~~~~

¾ cup strained fresh lime juice   5 cups cold water

16 packets calorie-free sugar substitute   1 lime, sliced

Stir together the lime juice, sweetener, and water. Add the lime slices, and pour over ice to serve. *Makes 6 servings. Amount per serving:* Calories 12, Fat 0.1 g, % calories from fat 7%. *Food group servings per serving:* Fruit 0.2.

RED ZINGER ICED TEA

~~~~~~~~~~~~~~~~~~~~~~~~~~~~~~~~~~~~~

6 Red Zinger tea bags   Calorie-free sugar substitute

4 cups boiling water   Orange slices for garnish

Brew the tea bags in the boiling water according to package directions. Stir in the sweetener to taste, and cool to room temperature. Pour over ice to serve. Garnish with the orange slices. *Makes 1 quart/4 servings. Amount per serving:* Calories 14, Fat 0 g, % calories from fat 0%. *Food group servings per serving:* None.

WHAT PARENTS SHOULD KNOW

Some parents worry that eating healthfully means spending more money on exotic health foods and special ingredients. You can save money and feed your family healthy foods if you do the following (based on a family of four):

- *Instead of expensive breakfast cereal, serve whole wheat toast spread with peanut butter or with a thin slice of cheese toasted on top.*

- *Make your own waffles with whole grain flour, and top them with fruit instead of butter and syrup. Store extra ones in the freezer for next time.*

- *Cook your own low-fat, whole-grain breakfast muffins.*

- *Make sandwiches with more lettuce, tomatoes, and vegetables and less meat.*

- *Make your own turkey breast and Swiss cheese sandwiches for your next picnic instead of buying them at the deli.*

- *Buy a quart of yogurt and dish it out into single servings instead of buying individual cups.*

- *Stock up on canned tuna (all white packed in water) on sale. Use tuna as a high-protein addition to salads and other dishes.*

- *Use hard-boiled eggs to add protein to your lunches.*

- *Cook with fiber-rich, low-fat lentils or other dried legumes, which are cheap and easy to use.*

- *Eliminate one meat dish per week and substitute a grain-based entrée.*

- *Buy pasta in bulk instead of in boxes.*

- *When making lasagna, substitute a box of frozen spinach (thawed) for half the cheeses. You'll save money and use less fat.*

- *Make your own tomato sauce. Simmer with onions, green peppers, and whatever you like.*

- *Buy fresh broccoli instead of frozen. Use the chopped stems for soups, pasta, salads or chili.*

- *Grate your own reduced-fat cheese instead of buying it already shredded.*

- *Make your own juice bars by freezing juice in paper cups.*

- *Buy potatoes in 5- or 10-pound bags.*

- *Drink water instead of other beverages, especially when eating out.*

- *Buy apples by the bag.*

Chapter 15

The Fit Legion

We'd like to change the way America eats and exercises, one family at a time. Your family is already part of the "Fit Legion." If you're limiting television and video games, encouraging active pastimes, exercising with your kids, keeping unhealthy or junk foods out of your pantry, stocking your shelves with healthy snacks, teaching and reinforcing portion control, praising your kids for the good work they're doing, encouraging them to participate in sports, watching the fat and sugar content of the foods you prepare, eating in restaurants less frequently and eating more wisely when you do, rewarding your child with things that make them active and not with food, helping them stay focused and motivated and setting the best example you can set, then in your own home you're helping to fight the obesity epidemic.

You can, however, do many things in your neighborhood, school district, town and state. There is the beginning of a new social movement afoot, but it needs all of us to keep it going. We have recognized that America has a weight problem. Books such as Marion Nestle's *Food Politics: How the Food Industry Influences Nutrition and Health,* Greg Critser's *Fat Land,* and Eric Schlosser's *Fast Food Nation* have raised America's consciousness about the ways the marketing and advertising of fast foods, snack foods, and other products full of fat, sugar, and salt have invaded our homes, schools, and workplaces.

In the schools, some communities have begun to recognize the need to restore physical education. Organizations such as P.E.4Life (www.pe4life.com) are setting up pilot programs, and the Department of Education offers grants to school districts to finance physical education. In many school districts, physical education is being redesigned with less emphasis on competitive, skill-based athletics and more on achieving personal fitness goals. Climbing walls and training circuits are being offered as alternatives to team sports.

"KidShape empowers the kids!"

—KidShape parent

In the courts, some lawyers are developing strategies to bring class action suits against companies who knowingly contribute to obesity.

In Congress, legislation has been proposed to levy a soda tax similar to the tax on cigarettes. Other lawmakers have suggested laws requiring more specific warning labels on foods high in salt or fat, or new taxes on unhealthy foods marketed specifically to kids. One Senate panel is discussing the Improved Nutrition and Physical Activity Act, a bill to authorize teaching better eating and exercise habits in our schools. Lawsuits are being brought against fast-food chains to require more truthful advertising.

All these initiatives need your support. Adults, parents, teachers, coaches, school nurses, and guidance counselors all have a role, and a responsibility, to make decisions about the curriculum in schools, the safety of neighborhoods, and the priorities of communities.

Specifically, what can you do?

GATHER INFORMATION. You can advocate for change in many ways. The first step is usually to gather as much information as possible. A good place is www.fitness.gov, where you will find many President's Council on Physical Fitness and Sports research digests. (You can access the Internet at public libraries if you don't have Internet access at home.) At the local level, you can find the curriculum requirements for physical education in your school district and see if your child's school is in compliance—state offices do not necessarily closely monitor this. Are all your kids' physical education instructors certified? Does your school have a policy for administering physical fitness tests? If so, is it giving them? And how do the results compare to the national average? Does your school evaluate students' health? Does it sell unhealthy foods in hallway vending machines?

ATTEND SCHOOL BOARD MEETINGS. In the past two decades, our nation's schools have been faced with the challenge of improving academic performance while cutting budgets. Something had to go, and that something has too often been physical education. In many schools gym classes only meet two or three days a week. Other schools offer only four- or six-week sessions. You have the right to ask for a real physical education program in your child's school, five days a week, kindergarten through 12th grade, taught by qualified physical education instructors.

CHECK OUT SCHOOL CAFETERIAS. At school board meetings, advocate for good nutrition in the cafeterias. Find out exactly what your child has been eating and measure the fat and sugar contents of the foods being served, as you did in your own home. If it isn't healthy, raise a fuss. Ask that your schools get rid of all the vending machines, and if that doesn't work, insist that those vending machines include healthy foods such as baked tortilla chips, nonfat popcorn, low-fat granola bars, trail mixes, dried or fresh fruits, low-fat yogurt, skim or nonfat milk, 100 percent fruit frozen bars, fig bars, or graham crackers. Lobby to get rid of the soda machines, and if your school district has subcontracted to fast-food chains, raise your voice in protest—insist that your child's school be free of junk food and soda.

ADVOCATE FOR NUTRITION EDUCATION. Ask that health classes include nutrition education as well as home economics, where your children can learn how to cook, what to cook, and how to shop for it on a budget. In many schools, home economics classes have been cut along with physical education classes. Ask that such classes start early, before bad habits become too entrenched. Ask that your child's school administer the President's Council on Physical Fitness and Sports Challenge test and send the results home along with students' report cards. Too many parents are in denial about their child's weight problem—receiving a health report will encourage them to take action.

HELP LIMIT TELEVISION. Support initiatives to limit television watching, including the PTA's annual Turn Your TV Off Week. Appeal directly to food companies, as well as television networks, and ask them not to advertise junk foods during children's programming.

TRY FOR JUNK FOOD TAX. Ask your congressional representatives to support a tax on junk food and sodas. What's truly needed is a new public health and education initiative that can be joined and followed by families and communities across the country. Such a nationwide movement hasn't been implemented since John F. Kennedy's Presidential Fitness Program of the early 1960s. A tax on junk foods and sodas would be a good start and a way to raise revenues to support physical education classes in our budget-strapped schools.

"The most valuable things our family learned were how to measure foods and how to use the calorie charts for fast-food restaurants."

—KidShape parent

LOBBY FOR INSURANCE HELP. Advocate to force your health providers to cover the costs of obesity prevention and treatment, which can include a referral to a dietary specialist. A first step is to appeal to your insurer's governing board.

INCREASE RECREATION AREAS. Work to increase the number of safe and accessible recreational areas in your community. This can mean anything from organizing park clean-up crews to forming citizen patrols, in addition to asking for an increased police presence and writing to your district representatives on your city council.

MAKE CONTACT. You can write letters to your school board members, superintendents, city councilmen, state education offices, members of Congress, and senators. If you include a petition signed by as many registered voters as possible, all the better. Send copies or press releases to the local newspapers and television stations. It might be even more effective if you visit your representatives in person, particularly if you're accompanied by a television crew and a dozen or so overweight kids in tow, asking for legislative action requiring increased gym classes or better nutritional education.

DO SOME ORGANIZING. Closer to home, if your school isn't providing adequate activities for your kids, do it yourself—organize outing clubs, sports teams, athletic competitions, hiking clubs, or other community sports outlets. Clear vacant lots and build skate parks or dirt bike parks. If you live where it's cold enough, make an ice skating rink in your backyard. Buy nets if your local basketball court needs them. Volunteer to coach teams at your local park. If your school physical education department is understaffed, volunteer to help out. Find like-minded adults with kids and organize camping or canoe trips.

Yes, all this will cost you time and some money, but it will cost more if your sedentary and overweight children develop serious diseases later on. And remember that it is costly for all of us when health resources are spent on diseases caused by being overweight. It is clearly in your own self-interest as an individual to work at the community level for social change.

WHAT PARENTS SHOULD KNOW

The good news is that things are changing—and it's because of consumers like you. Food companies respond to the pressures of the marketplace, and more pressure is being put on food companies to offer healthy products. In July 2003, Kraft Foods announced its intention to reduce the fat and sugar contents of some of their products, reduce portion sizes, and cease marketing its products in schools. Frito-Lay, Kraft's chief competitor, has said it will remove trans-fatty acids (which can clog arteries) from its snack foods.

The fast-food chains that once vended their burgers in nonbiodegradable Styrofoam containers switched to recyclable paper when consumers demanded it.

Similarly, in 1990, in response to the public's health concerns, McDonald's switched from frying potatoes in beef tallow and cottonseed oil to pure vegetable oil. It is exactly those kinds of market pressures that generate change. The potato and fast-food industries are already trying to develop more healthful ways to cook French fries, using better oils without the trans-fatty acids that add extra calories.

The food industry wants to give us what we want. It's simply up to us to tell them. If we change what we want, they'll change what they give us.

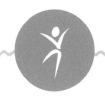

Appendix 1

Materials to Photocopy for Journals and Workshops

Before you begin the program, you should photocopy the materials in this section. Alternatively, you can print larger size versions (8½ x 11 inches) from the KidShape Web site at www.kidshape.com. The quantities given for the weekly forms are guidelines only, based on completing the workshops in seven weeks. If your family takes longer, you will need additional copies of the weekly materials. You may also need additional copies of the Weekly Food Log "continued" pages as you proceed through the program.

Forms	Number of copies
Weekly Food Log	6 copies per participant
Weekly Food Log, *continued*	12 copies per participant
Weekly Activity Log	6 copies per participant
Weekly Goals	6 copies per participant
Weekly Journal Page: Child	6 copies per child

KiDShape

Forms	Number of copies
Weekly Journal Page: Adult	6 copies per adult
Weekly Point Chart	1 copy per participant
Family Reward Chart	1 copy
The Contract (The First Meeting)	1 copy per participant
Information Survey (The First Meeting and Workshop 7)	1 copy per participant
Body Mass Index-for-Age Percentiles: Boys (The First Meeting and Workshop 7)	1 copy per boy
Stature-for-Age and Weight-for-Age Percentiles: Boys (The First Meeting and Workshop 7)	1 copy per boy
Body Mass Index-for-Age Percentiles: Girls (The First Meeting and Workshop 7)	1 copy per girl
Stature-for-Age and Weight-for-Age Percentiles: Girls (The First Meeting and Workshop 7)	1 copy per girl
Body Mass Index Table: Adults (The First Meeting and Workshop 7)	1 copy per adult
Your Personal Food and Fitness Survey (Workshops 1 and 7)	2 copies per participant
Blank Pyramid (Workshops 1 and 3)	3 copies per participant (optional)
My Daily Food Guide Pyramid (Workshop 3)	1 copy per participant

Food Cards (Workshop 3)   Instructions: Make enough
copies of each food group card for each participant. It is a good idea to use a
different color paper for each food group. (If you have access to a color printer,
you can print out the cards in color from www.kidshape.com.) Since there are
four copies of each card on a sheet of paper, for a team of two adults and two
children, make the following number of copies (adjust the quantities as necessary to suit your family size):

Food group	Sheet color	Number of copies
Grains	Yellow	8
Vegetables	Green	4
Fruit	Orange	3
Milk, Yogurt	Blue	3
Protein	Red	3
Fats, Sweets	Pink	6

Forms	Number of copies
Family Meal Plan (Workshop 3)	1 copy
Body Image Survey (Workshop 4)	1 copy per participant

WEEKLY FOOD LOG

WEEK OF _____

Write down each item you eat or drink every day, including the date and the time you ate the item, as well as how much you ate. Next write down your hunger level before you consumed it, and your hunger level afterward. Use the hunger scale below:

Starving	Really hungry	Hungry	Hungry on and off	A little hungry	Not hungry at all	Satisfied	Full	Stuffed	Sick
1	2	3	4	5	6	7	8	9	10

In the last column, write down any feelings before and after eating. Are you bored, angry, upset, or experiencing some other feeling? If so, write such feelings down.

Date	Time	Food or drink	Amount	Hunger	Feelings
				/	
				/	
				/	
				/	
				/	
				/	
				/	
				/	
				/	
				/	
				/	
				/	
				/	
				/	
				/	

WEEKLY FOOD LOG. *continued*

WEEK OF _____

Date	Time	Food or drink	Amount	Hunger	Feelings
				/	
				/	
				/	
				/	
				/	
				/	
				/	
				/	
				/	
				/	
				/	
				/	
				/	
				/	
				/	
				/	
				/	
				/	
				/	
				/	
				/	
				/	
				/	
				/	
				/	
				/	
				/	
				/	

WEEKLY ACTIVITY LOG

WEEK OF _____

For each day you complete the indicated physical activity for at least 30 minutes, put a check in the box.

Activity	Sun.	Mon.	Tues.	Wed.	Thurs.	Fri.	Sat.
Walking							
Running							
Actively playing at park							
Riding bicycle							
Dancing							
Playing sports like basketball or soccer							
Jumping rope, nonstop							
Exercise video							
Other:							

WEEKLY GOALS

WEEK OF _____

The first step toward achieving goals is to write them down. Write down two goals related to the way you eat and two related to the way you are physically active.

My goals for this week are . . .

I am in charge of what I eat. This week I will do the following:

1. _____
_____

2. _____
_____

I am in charge of my physical activity. This week I will do the following:

3. _____
_____

4. _____
_____

Goal Tracking

For each day you meet your goal that you have written above, put a sticker in the box. This will help you keep track of meeting your goals.

Goals	Sun.	Mon.	Tues.	Wed.	Thurs.	Fri.	Sat.
Goal 1							
Goal 2							
Goal 3							
Goal 4							

WEEKLY JOURNAL PAGE: CHILD

WEEK OF _____

Use the following scale to answer the questions:

Great	Okay	So-so	Could be better	Not great
1	2	3	4	5

	Sun.	Mon.	Tues.	Wed.	Thurs.	Fri.	Sat.
How was my eating today?							
How was my exercise today?							
How did I feel today?							

Name one good thing that happened today.

Sun. _____

Mon. _____

Tues. _____

Wed. _____

Thurs. _____

Fri. _____

Sat. _____

My thoughts:

Sun. _____
_____

Mon. _____
_____

Tues. _____
_____

Wed. _____
_____

Thurs. _____
_____

Fri. _____
_____

Sat. _____
_____

WEEKLY JOURNAL PAGE: ADULT

WEEK OF _____

Use the following scale to answer the questions:

Great	Okay	So-so	Could be better	Not great
1	2	3	4	5

	Sun.	Mon.	Tues.	Wed.	Thurs.	Fri.	Sat.
How was my eating today?							
How was my child(ren)'s eating today?							
How was my exercise today?							
How was my child(ren)'s exercise today?							
How did I feel today?							
How did my child(ren) feel today?							

Name one good thing that happened today.

Sun. _____

Mon. _____

Tues. _____

Wed. _____

Thurs. _____

Fri. _____

Sat. _____

My thoughts:

Sun. _____
_____

Mon. _____
_____

Tues. _____
_____

Wed. _____
_____

Thurs. _____
_____

Fri. _____
_____

Sat. _____
_____

WEEKLY POINT CHART

At each workshop, mark down 10 points for attending the workshop. Then for each task you accomplished in the previous week, write 10 points in the box. Add any additional points at the bottom.

	Workshop 1	Workshop 2	Workshop 3	Workshop 4	Workshop 5	Workshop 6	Workshop 7
Attending the workshop							
Completing the Weekly Food Log							
Completing the Weekly Activity Log							
Completing the Weekly Goals							
Completing the Weekly Journal Page (for at least four days)							
Additional points							
Workshop TOTAL							

FAMILY REWARD CHART

Fill in the names of family members in the top row and then track their weekly points in the boxes below. Subtract the point value of any awards received and indicate what the reward was.

Name of family member:					
Workshop 1 points value					
Subtract cashed-in points					
Total points at end of Workshop 1					
Workshop 2 points value					
Plus total points at end of Workshop 1					
Subtract cashed-in points					
Total points at end of Workshop 2					
Workshop 3 points value					
Plus total points at end of Workshop 2					
Subtract cashed-in points					
Total points at end of Workshop 3					
Workshop 4 points value					
Plus total points at end of Workshop 3					
Subtract cashed-in points					
Total points at end of Workshop 4					
Workshop 5 points value					
Plus total points at end of Workshop 4					
Subtract cashed-in points					
Total points at end of Workshop 5					
Workshop 6 points value					
Plus total points at end of Workshop 5					
Subtract cashed-in points					
Total points at end of Workshop 6					
Workshop 7 points value					
Plus total points at end of Workshop 6					
Subtract cashed-in points					
Total points at end of Workshop 7					

THE CONTRACT (The First Meeting)

I will respect everyone else's *privacy*. There is to be no prying. Each individual has the right to decide whether to share private thoughts during family meetings or discussions. Anybody who wants to simply sit and listen may do so, with the understanding that participation is beneficial but voluntary.

I will show everyone *respect*. There will be no teasing and no scolding. The idea is for the whole team to arrive at its goals, but each individual will progress at a different rate.

I will uphold the family *confidentiality*. There will be no telling. What happens and what is said within the family stays within the family. Participating in a weight loss and fitness program is not a secret or something to be ashamed of, but family members should feel free to discuss their thoughts and feelings knowing they need not feel bashful or shy, or worry that friends or people outside the family will find out things they'd rather keep private.

I will *trust* my family members. There will be no blaming, and no lying. I promise to make my best effort to be honest, accepting that no one is perfect and everyone makes mistakes from time to time.

I will show up *on time* for family workshops once a week.

I will eat *together* with my family *at least* five times a week.

I will show up on time, dressed appropriately, to *exercise* with my family at least three times a week for 30 minutes.

I will complete *all* my homework assignments.

I will *listen* to others without interrupting.

I will be *positive* and try to encourage everyone in my family.

If you agree to all of the above, sign below.

_____   _____

Your name   Date

INFORMATION SURVEY (The First Meeting and Workshop 7)

1. Why are you choosing to start the KidShape program?

_____

_____

2. Whose idea was it to start the program?

_____

_____

3. Have you tried to eat healthier or exercise more before?   YES / NO

4. If yes, how many times have you tried?   1 / 2 / 3 / 4 / MORE

5. What changes do you hope to make as a result of the KidShape program?

_____

_____

6. Do you think it will be easy or hard to make changes?   EASY / HARD / VERY HARD

7. What changes do you think will be hardest for you to make?

_____ Eat fewer sweets	_____ Eat fewer fatty foods
_____ Watch less TV	_____ Eat more vegetables
_____ Drink less soda	_____ Play fewer video/computer games
_____ Exercise more	_____ Other: _____

8. Do you think that you are overweight?   YES / NO

9. Are you teased about your weight?   NEVER / SOMETIMES / OFTEN

10. If yes, who teases you?   PARENT / BROTHER / SISTER / KIDS AT SCHOOL / OTHER: _____

11. What are three of your best qualities?   1) _____   2) _____   3) _____

RESULTS OF FITNESS TEST

	The First Meeting	Workshop 7
Part 1: Curl-ups		
Part 2: Push-ups		
Part 3: V-sit reach		
Part 4: Endurance walk/run		
Part 5: Pull-ups		
Part 6: Shuttle run		

BODY MASS INDEX-FOR-AGE PERCENTILES: BOYS, 2 to 20 YEARS
(The First Meeting and Workshop 7)

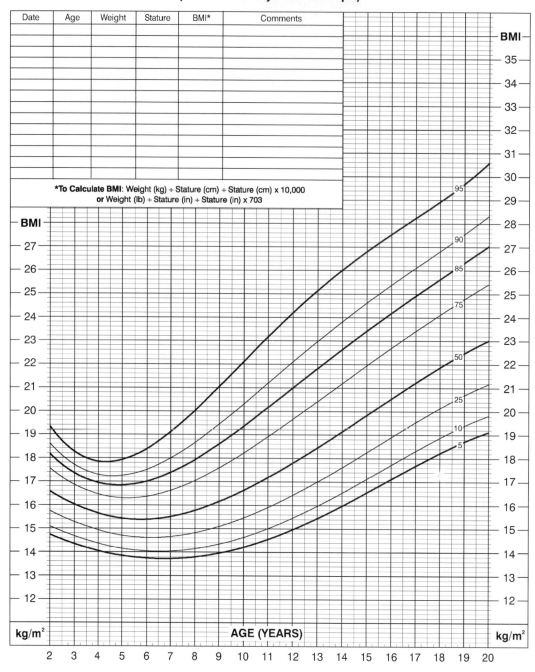

Date	Age	Weight	Stature	BMI*	Comments

*To Calculate BMI: Weight (kg) ÷ Stature (cm) ÷ Stature (cm) x 10,000
or Weight (lb) ÷ Stature (in) ÷ Stature (in) x 703

AGE (YEARS)

Published May 30, 2000 (modified 10/16/00).
SOURCE: Developed by the National Center for Health Statistics in collaboration with
the National Center for Chronic Disease Prevention and Health Promotion (2000).
http://www.cdc.gov/growthcharts

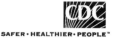

SAFER · HEALTHIER · PEOPLE™

Source: Center for Disease Control.

STATURE-FOR-AGE AND WEIGHT-FOR-AGE PERCENTILES: BOYS, 2 to 20 YEARS
(The First Meeting and Workshop 7)

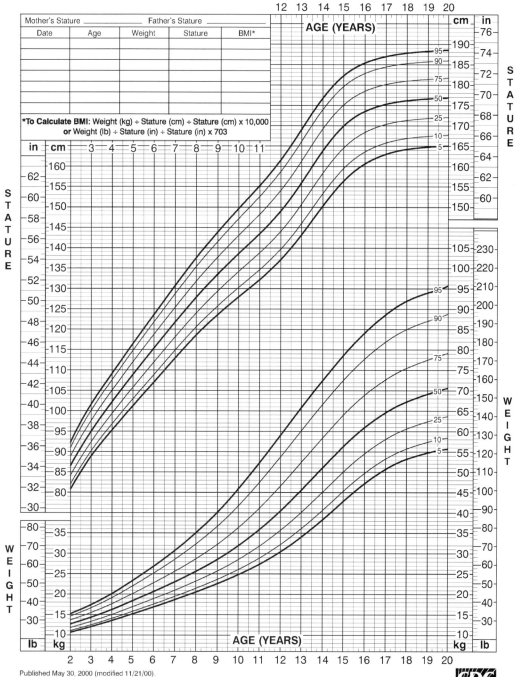

Published May 30, 2000 (modified 11/21/00).
SOURCE: Developed by the National Center for Health Statistics in collaboration with
the National Center for Chronic Disease Prevention and Health Promotion (2000).
http://www.cdc.gov/growthcharts

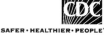

SAFER·HEALTHIER·PEOPLE™

Source: Center for Disease Control.

227

BODY MASS INDEX-FOR-AGE PERCENTILES: GIRLS, 2 to 20 YEARS
(The First Meeting and Workshop 7)

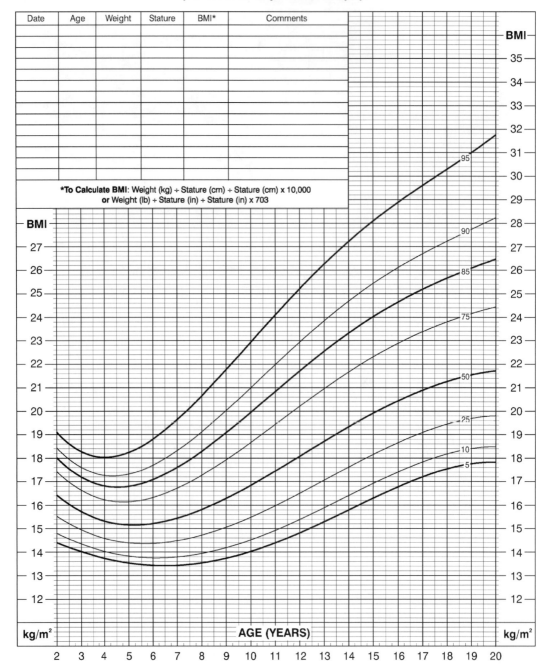

*To Calculate BMI: Weight (kg) ÷ Stature (cm) ÷ Stature (cm) x 10,000
or Weight (lb) ÷ Stature (in) ÷ Stature (in) x 703

Date	Age	Weight	Stature	BMI*	Comments

Published May 30, 2000 (modified 10/16/00).
SOURCE: Developed by the National Center for Health Statistics in collaboration with
the National Center for Chronic Disease Prevention and Health Promotion (2000).
http://www.cdc.gov/growthcharts

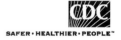

SAFER · HEALTHIER · PEOPLE™

Source: Center for Disease Control.

STATURE-FOR-AGE AND WEIGHT-FOR-AGE PERCENTILES: GIRLS, 2 to 20 YEARS
(The First Meeting and Workshop 7)

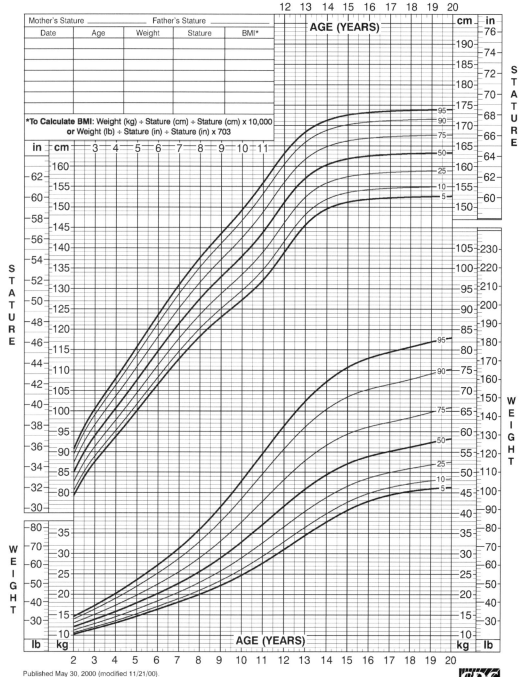

Mother's Stature _____ Father's Stature _____

Date	Age	Weight	Stature	BMI*

*To Calculate BMI: Weight (kg) ÷ Stature (cm) ÷ Stature (cm) x 10,000
or Weight (lb) ÷ Stature (in) ÷ Stature (in) x 703

AGE (YEARS)

STATURE

WEIGHT

Published May 30, 2000 (modified 11/21/00).
SOURCE: Developed by the National Center for Health Statistics in collaboration with
the National Center for Chronic Disease Prevention and Health Promotion (2000).
http://www.cdc.gov/growthcharts

SAFER · HEALTHIER · PEOPLE™

Source: Center for Disease Control.

BODY MASS INDEX TABLE: ADULTS
(The First Meeting and Workshop 7)

Date	Age	Weight	Stature	BMI

Body Weight (pounds)

Height (inches)	Normal 19	20	21	22	23	24	Overweight 25	26	27	28	29	Obese 30	31	32	33	34	35	36	37	38	39	Extreme Obesity 40	41	42	43	44	45	46	47	48	49	50	51	52	53	54
58	91	96	100	105	110	115	119	124	129	134	138	143	148	153	158	162	167	172	177	181	186	191	196	201	205	210	215	220	224	229	234	239	244	248	253	258
59	94	99	104	109	114	119	124	128	133	138	143	148	153	158	163	168	173	178	183	188	193	198	203	208	212	217	222	227	232	237	242	247	252	257	262	267
60	97	102	107	112	118	123	128	133	138	143	148	153	158	163	168	174	179	184	189	194	199	204	209	215	220	225	230	235	240	245	250	255	261	266	271	276
61	100	106	111	116	122	127	132	137	143	148	153	158	164	169	174	180	185	190	195	201	206	211	217	222	227	232	238	243	248	254	259	264	269	275	280	285
62	104	109	115	120	126	131	136	142	147	153	158	164	169	175	180	186	191	196	202	207	213	218	224	229	235	240	246	251	256	262	267	273	278	284	289	295
63	107	113	118	124	130	135	141	146	152	158	163	169	175	180	186	191	197	203	208	214	220	225	231	237	242	248	254	259	265	270	278	282	287	293	299	304
64	110	116	122	128	134	140	145	151	157	163	169	174	180	186	192	197	204	209	215	221	227	232	238	244	250	256	262	267	273	279	285	291	296	302	308	314
65	114	120	126	132	138	144	150	156	162	168	174	180	186	192	198	204	210	216	222	228	234	240	246	252	258	264	270	276	282	288	294	300	306	312	318	324
66	118	124	130	136	142	148	155	161	167	173	179	186	192	198	204	210	216	223	229	235	241	247	253	260	266	272	278	284	291	297	303	309	315	322	328	334
67	121	127	134	140	146	153	159	166	172	178	185	191	198	204	211	217	223	230	236	242	249	255	261	268	274	280	287	293	299	306	312	319	325	331	338	344
68	125	131	138	144	151	158	164	171	177	184	190	197	203	210	216	223	230	236	243	249	256	262	269	276	282	289	295	302	308	315	322	328	335	341	348	354
69	128	135	142	149	155	162	169	176	182	189	196	203	209	216	223	230	236	243	250	257	263	270	277	284	291	297	304	311	318	324	331	338	345	351	358	365
70	132	139	146	153	160	167	174	181	188	195	202	209	216	222	229	236	243	250	257	264	271	278	285	292	299	306	313	320	327	334	341	348	355	362	369	376
71	136	143	150	157	165	172	179	186	193	200	208	215	222	229	236	243	250	257	265	272	279	286	293	301	308	315	322	329	338	343	351	358	365	372	379	386
72	140	147	154	162	169	177	184	191	199	206	213	221	228	235	242	250	258	265	272	279	287	294	302	309	316	324	331	338	346	353	361	368	375	383	390	397
73	144	151	159	166	174	182	189	197	204	212	219	227	235	242	250	257	265	272	280	288	295	302	310	318	325	333	340	348	355	363	371	378	386	393	401	408
74	148	155	163	171	179	186	194	202	210	218	225	233	241	249	256	264	272	280	287	295	303	311	319	326	334	342	350	358	365	373	381	389	396	404	412	420
75	152	160	168	176	184	192	200	208	216	224	232	240	248	256	264	272	279	287	295	303	311	319	327	335	343	351	359	367	375	383	391	399	407	415	423	431
76	156	164	172	180	189	197	205	213	221	230	238	246	254	263	271	279	287	295	304	312	320	328	336	344	353	361	369	377	385	394	402	410	418	426	435	443

Source: Adapted from *Clinical Guidelines on the Identification, Evaluation, and Treatment of Overweight and Obesity in Adults: The Evidence Report.*

Source: National Institutes of Health.

YOUR PERSONAL FOOD AND FITNESS SURVEY (Workshops 1 and 7)

FOODS

1. How many times a day do you eat

Vegetables? ___

Fruit? ___

High-fat foods (such as French fries or chips)? ___

Sugary foods (cookies, candy)? ___

2. How many times per week does your family eat out (takeout, fast-food places, restaurants)? ____

3. At which restaurants does your family usually eat?

_____

_____

DRINKS

4. How many times per day do you drink

100 percent fruit juice? ___

Other fruit drinks (such as Capri Sun, Fruit Punch)? ___

Milk? Whole, low-fat, or nonfat?_____

Chocolate milk? ____

Soda? Diet or regular? _____

ACTIVITIES

5. How many hours per day do you

Watch TV? ___

Play video games? ___

Use a computer? ___

6. How many days per week

Do you participate in school physical education? ___

Are you physically active after school? ___

7. How many minutes are you active each day (doing things such as playing tag, riding a bike, sports)

In physical education at school? ___

After school? ___

Weekend days? ___

8. What activities do you participate in on weekends?

_____

_____

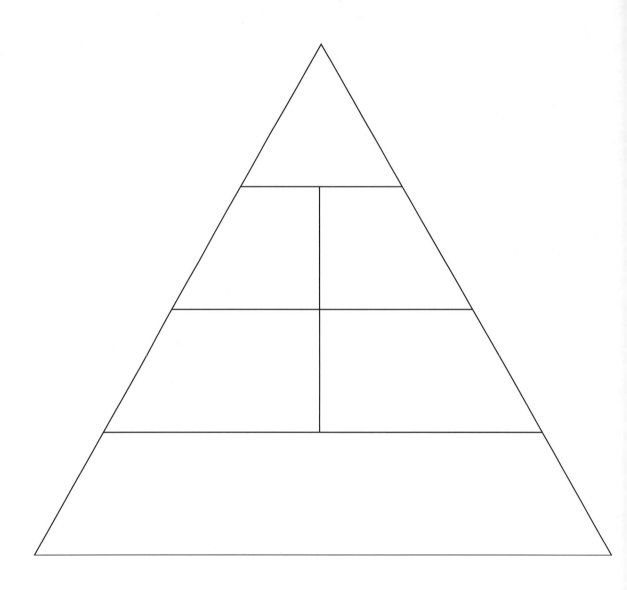

MY DAILY FOOD GUIDE PYRAMID (Workshop 3)

Using Table 7.2, fill in the correct number of servings for each food group to create your own personal food guide pyramid.

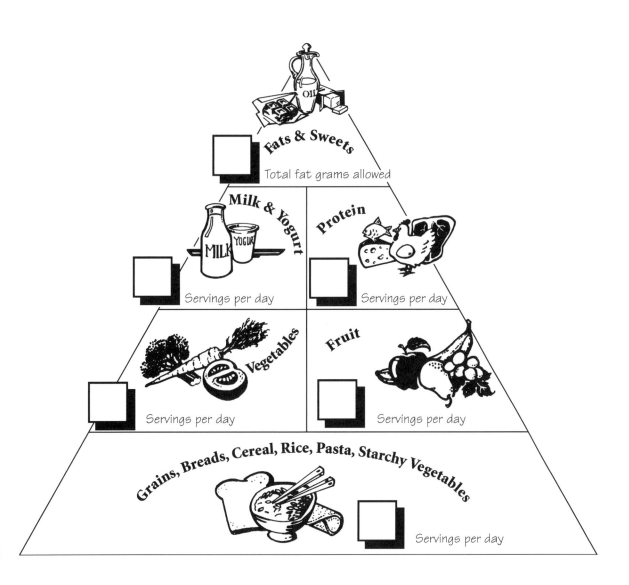

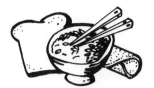

ONE SERVING **1**

- 1 slice of bread or ½ English muffin/bun
- ¾ cup dry, unsweetened cereal or ½ cup frosted cereal
- ½ cup cooked cereal
- ½ cup cooked rice, pasta, corn, peas, or mashed potato
- 1 small baked or boiled potato
- 3 cups popcorn (popped, no fat added or low-fat microwave)
- 1 (6-inch) corn tortilla or 1 (7- to 8-inch) flour tortilla
- 1 waffle, 4½-inch square, reduced fat
- 5 or 6 small crackers, low-fat

GRAINS
BREAD, CEREAL, RICE, PASTA, STARCHY VEGETABLES

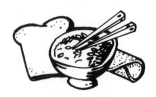

ONE SERVING **1**

- 1 slice of bread or ½ English muffin/bun
- ¾ cup dry, unsweetened cereal or ½ cup frosted cereal
- ½ cup cooked cereal
- ½ cup cooked rice, pasta, corn, peas, or mashed potato
- 1 small baked or boiled potato
- 3 cups popcorn (popped, no fat added or low-fat microwave)
- 1 (6-inch) corn tortilla or 1 (7- to 8-inch) flour tortilla
- 1 waffle, 4½-inch square, reduced fat
- 5 or 6 small crackers, low-fat

GRAINS
BREAD, CEREAL, RICE, PASTA, STARCHY VEGETABLES

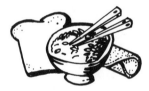

ONE SERVING **1**

- 1 slice of bread or ½ English muffin/bun
- ¾ cup dry, unsweetened cereal or ½ cup frosted cereal
- ½ cup cooked cereal
- ½ cup cooked rice, pasta, corn, peas, or mashed potato
- 1 small baked or boiled potato
- 3 cups popcorn (popped, no fat added or low-fat microwave)
- 1 (6-inch) corn tortilla or 1 (7- to 8-inch) flour tortilla
- 1 waffle, 4½-inch square, reduced fat
- 5 or 6 small crackers, low-fat

GRAINS
BREAD, CEREAL, RICE, PASTA, STARCHY VEGETABLES

ONE SERVING **1**

- 1 slice of bread or ½ English muffin/bun
- ¾ cup dry, unsweetened cereal or ½ cup frosted cereal
- ½ cup cooked cereal
- ½ cup cooked rice, pasta, corn, peas, or mashed potato
- 1 small baked or boiled potato
- 3 cups popcorn (popped, no fat added or low-fat microwave)
- 1 (6-inch) corn tortilla or 1 (7- to 8-inch) flour tortilla
- 1 waffle, 4½-inch square, reduced fat
- 5 or 6 small crackers, low-fat

GRAINS
BREAD, CEREAL, RICE, PASTA, STARCHY VEGETABLES

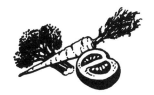

ONE SERVING 1

• 1 cup raw vegetables

• ½ cup cooked vegetables

• ½ cup tomato or vegetable juice

• ½ cup tomato sauce

VEGETABLES

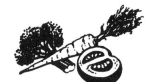

ONE SERVING 1

• 1 cup raw vegetables

• ½ cup cooked vegetables

• ½ cup tomato or vegetable juice

• ½ cup tomato sauce

VEGETABLES

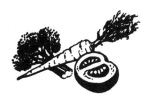

ONE SERVING 1

• 1 cup raw vegetables

• ½ cup cooked vegetables

• ½ cup tomato or vegetable juice

• ½ cup tomato sauce

VEGETABLES

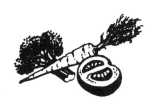

ONE SERVING 1

• 1 cup raw vegetables

• ½ cup cooked vegetables

• ½ cup tomato or vegetable juice

• ½ cup tomato sauce

VEGETABLES

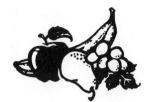

- 1 small fresh fruit
- ½ cup canned fruit (canned in water, juice, or extra light syrup)
- ¼ cup dried fruit
- ½ cup 100% fruit juice
- ½ (9-inch) banana
- 16 grapes
- 1 (100% fruit juice) frozen bar

FRUIT

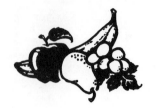

- 1 small fresh fruit
- ½ cup canned fruit (canned in water, juice, or extra light syrup)
- ¼ cup dried fruit
- ½ cup 100% fruit juice
- ½ (9-inch) banana
- 16 grapes
- 1 (100% fruit juice) frozen bar

FRUIT

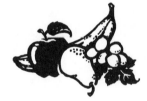

- 1 small fresh fruit
- ½ cup canned fruit (canned in water, juice, or extra light syrup)
- ¼ cup dried fruit
- ½ cup 100% fruit juice
- ½ (9-inch) banana
- 16 grapes
- 1 (100% fruit juice) frozen bar

FRUIT

- 1 small fresh fruit
- ½ cup canned fruit (canned in water, juice, or extra light syrup)
- ¼ cup dried fruit
- ½ cup 100% fruit juice
- ½ (9-inch) banana
- 16 grapes
- 1 (100% fruit juice) frozen bar

FRUIT

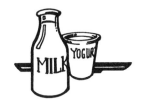

ONE SERVING 1

- 1 cup skim, ½% fat, or 1% fat milk

- 1 cup low-fat or nonfat yogurt

- 1 cup nonfat or low-fat buttermilk

- ⅓ cup nonfat dry milk

- ½ cup evaporated skim milk

MILK, YOGURT

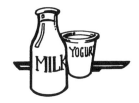

ONE SERVING 1

- 1 cup skim, ½% fat, or 1% fat milk

- 1 cup low-fat or nonfat yogurt

- 1 cup nonfat or low-fat buttermilk

- ⅓ cup nonfat dry milk

- ½ cup evaporated skim milk

MILK, YOGURT

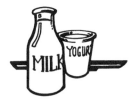

ONE SERVING 1

- 1 cup skim, ½% fat, or 1% fat milk

- 1 cup low-fat or nonfat yogurt

- 1 cup nonfat or low-fat buttermilk

- ⅓ cup nonfat dry milk

- ½ cup evaporated skim milk

MILK, YOGURT

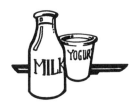

ONE SERVING 1

- 1 cup skim, ½% fat, or 1% fat milk

- 1 cup low-fat or nonfat yogurt

- 1 cup nonfat or low-fat buttermilk

- ⅓ cup nonfat dry milk

- ½ cup evaporated skim milk

MILK, YOGURT

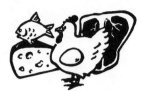

ONE SERVING **1**

- 1 ounce cooked lean meat, poultry, fish, or shellfish
- 1 egg or 2 egg whites
- ½ cup cooked beans or lentils
- 1 ounce low-fat cheese
- ½ to ¾ cup tuna, canned in water
- ½ to ¾ cup low-fat or nonfat cottage cheese
- 2 tablespoons natural peanut butter (= 1 oz. protein + 1 fat)
- 10 peanuts

PROTEIN

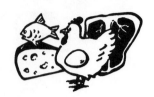

ONE SERVING **1**

- 1 ounce cooked lean meat, poultry, fish, or shellfish
- 1 egg or 2 egg whites
- ½ cup cooked beans or lentils
- 1 ounce low-fat cheese
- ½ to ¾ cup tuna, canned in water
- ½ to ¾ cup low-fat or nonfat cottage cheese
- 2 tablespoons natural peanut butter (= 1 oz. protein + 1 fat)
- 10 peanuts

PROTEIN

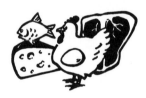

ONE SERVING **1**

- 1 ounce cooked lean meat, poultry, fish, or shellfish
- 1 egg or 2 egg whites
- ½ cup cooked beans or lentils
- 1 ounce low-fat cheese
- ½ to ¾ cup tuna, canned in water
- ½ to ¾ cup low-fat or nonfat cottage cheese
- 2 tablespoons natural peanut butter (= 1 oz. protein + 1 fat)
- 10 peanuts

PROTEIN

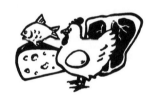

ONE SERVING **1**

- 1 ounce cooked lean meat, poultry, fish, or shellfish
- 1 egg or 2 egg whites
- ½ cup cooked beans or lentils
- 1 ounce low-fat cheese
- ½ to ¾ cup tuna, canned in water
- ½ to ¾ cup low-fat or nonfat cottage cheese
- 2 tablespoons natural peanut butter (= 1 oz. protein + 1 fat)
- 10 peanuts

PROTEIN

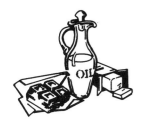

ONE
SERVING
1

- 1 teaspoon butter, margarine, oil, or mayonnaise
- 1 tablespoon reduced-fat butter, margarine, or mayonnaise
- 1 tablespoon cream cheese or salad dressing
- 2 tablespoons reduced-fat cream cheese or salad dressing
- 2 small cookies
- ½ cup light or reduced-fat ice cream or ¼ cup ice cream

FATS, SWEETS

USE SPARINGLY

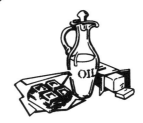

ONE
SERVING
1

- 1 teaspoon butter, margarine, oil, or mayonnaise
- 1 tablespoon reduced-fat butter, margarine, or mayonnaise
- 1 tablespoon cream cheese or salad dressing
- 2 tablespoons reduced-fat cream cheese or salad dressing
- 2 small cookies
- ½ cup light or reduced-fat ice cream or ¼ cup ice cream

FATS, SWEETS

USE SPARINGLY

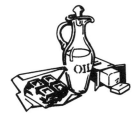

ONE
SERVING
1

- 1 teaspoon butter, margarine, oil, or mayonnaise
- 1 tablespoon reduced-fat butter, margarine, or mayonnaise
- 1 tablespoon cream cheese or salad dressing
- 2 tablespoons reduced-fat cream cheese or salad dressing
- 2 small cookies
- ½ cup light or reduced-fat ice cream or ¼ cup ice cream

FATS, SWEETS

USE SPARINGLY

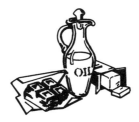

ONE
SERVING
1

- 1 teaspoon butter, margarine, oil, or mayonnaise
- 1 tablespoon reduced-fat butter, margarine, or mayonnaise
- 1 tablespoon cream cheese or salad dressing
- 2 tablespoons reduced-fat cream cheese or salad dressing
- 2 small cookies
- ½ cup light or reduced-fat ice cream or ¼ cup ice cream

FATS, SWEETS

USE SPARINGLY

FAMILY MEAL PLAN (Workshop 3)

Write down a sample menu for an entire day, putting a check in the corresponding boxes to designate the number of servings in each food group that your meal contains. Once you complete your menu for the day, count up each of your check marks for each food group. The check marks in each food group should equal the number of servings listed on your personal meal plan and the number of cards for your daily allowance.

Meals/Snacks	Breads/ Grains	Fruit	Vegetables	Milk/ Yogurt	Protein	Fats/ Sweets
Breakfast *Example:* *¾ cup Cheerios* *with 1 cup 1% milk,* *½ banana*	✔	✔		✔		
Snack						
Lunch						
Snack						
Dinner						
Snack						
TOTAL						

BODY IMAGE SURVEY (Workshop 4)

1. Three things I like about myself are

    A. _____

    B. _____

    C. _____

2. Three things I like about my body are

    A. _____

    B. _____

    C. _____

3. Three things I don't like about myself are

    A. _____

    B. _____

    C. _____

4. Three things I don't like about my body are

    A. _____

    B. _____

    C. _____

5. Of the things I don't like about myself or my body, which can be changed?

_____

_____

6. Of those things that are possible to change, which will I change?

_____

_____

7. Of those things that are not possible to change, which will I accept?

_____

_____

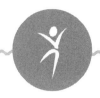

APPENDIX 2

Reference Materials

→ Vitamins and Minerals

→ Carry-Along Fast-Food Tables

→ Organizations That Can Help

VITAMINS AND MINERALS

Vitamin	Effect	Good sources
Water-soluble vitamins		
Thiamin (vitamin B1)	Promotes carbohydrate metabolism; needed for normal appetite, digestion, nerve function; enhances energy.	Pork, seafood, fortified grains, cereal.
Riboflavin (vitamin B2)	Needed for all food metabolism, maintains mucous membranes, helps maintain vision, helps release energy to cells.	Organ meats, beef, lamb, poultry, dark meat, dairy foods, fortified cereals, grains, dark green leafy vegetables.
Niacin/nicotinic acid (vitamin B3)	Needed in many enzymes that convert food to energy, promotes normal appetite and digestion, promotes nerve function.	Poultry, seafood, seeds, nuts, peanuts, potatoes, fortified whole-grain breads and cereals.
Pantothenic acid (vitamin B5)	Needed to break down food into molecular forms required by body; involved in making adrenal hormones and chemicals that regulate nerve function.	Found in almost all plant and animal foods.
Pyridoxine (vitamin B6)	Required for metabolism and absorption of protein, important in carbohydrate metabolism, helps form red blood cells, promotes nerve function.	Meats, fish, poultry, grains, cereals, spinach, sweet and white potatoes, bananas, prunes, watermelon.
Vitamin B12 (cobalamin)	Helps build genetic material (nucleic acid) required by all cells, helps form red blood cells.	All foods of animal origin, including meats, poultry, eggs, seafood, dairy foods.
Biotin, a B vitamin	Required for glucose metabolism and formation of certain fatty acids; plays an essential part in many bodily processes.	Produced by intestinal bacteria. Also obtained from meats, poultry, fish, eggs, nuts, seeds, legumes, vegetables.
Folic Acid (folate, folacin) a B vitamin	Needed to make genetic material (DNA, RNA); needed for making red blood cells.	Poultry, liver, dark green leafy vegetables, legumes, fortified whole-grain breads, cereals; oranges, grapefruit.
Vitamin C (ascorbic acid)	Helps bind cells together, strengthens blood vessel walls, may have antihistaminic effect against common cold symptoms.	Citrus fruits; strawberries, cantaloupe, watermelon, sweet potatoes, cabbage, cauliflower, broccoli, plantains, snow peas.

Fat-soluble vitamins	Effect	Good sources
Vitamin A	Keeps skin, hair, nails healthy; helps maintain gums, glands, bones, teeth; helps prevent infection; promotes eye function; prevents night blindness.	Milk and dairy foods; fortified cereals, green and yellow vegetables, deep yellow or orange fruits, organ meats.
Vitamin D	Helps build and maintain bones; needed for calcium absorption.	Egg yolks, fish oils, fortified milk and butter, exposure to sunlight without sunscreen.
Vitamin E	Helps form red blood cells, muscles, other tissues; antioxidant; stabilizes cell membranes; preserves fatty acids.	Poultry, seafood, green leafy vegetables, wheat germ, whole grains, seeds, nuts, butter, liver, egg yolk.
Vitamin K	Needed for normal blood clotting; helps maintain healthy bones.	Produced by intestinal bacteria, cow's milk, green leafy vegetables, pork, liver, oats, wheat, bran, whole grain.
Minerals		
Calcium	Builds bones, teeth; promotes nerve and muscle function; helps blood clot; helps activate enzymes that convert food into energy.	Milk and dairy foods, canned fish (salmon, sardines) with bones; oysters, broccoli, tofu (bean curd).
Chloride	Helps maintain acid-base balance of body fluids; component of hydrochloric acid in gastric juices needed for digestion.	Salt, processed foods, milk, water in some areas.
Chromium	Works with insulin in glucose metabolism.	Whole-grain breads and cereals, brewers yeast; peanuts.
Copper	Component of several enzymes, including one needed to make body's pigments; stimulates iron absorption; needed to make red blood cells, connective tissue, nerve fibers.	Nuts, dried peas, beans, barley, prunes, organ meats, lobster.
Fluoride	Promotes strong teeth and bones, especially in children; enhances body's uptake of calcium.	Fluoridated water, food cooked in fluoridated water, tea made with fluoridated water.
Iodine	Essential for function of thyroid gland.	Iodized salt, seafood, vegetables grown in iodine-rich soil.
Iron	Essential to make hemoglobin, the red oxygen-carrying pigment in blood, and myoglobin, a pigment that stores oxygen in muscles.	Red meat, liver, fish, shellfish, legumes, fortified breads, cereals, dried apricots.

Minerals *(continued)*	Effect	Good sources
Magnesium	Activates enzymes needed to release energy in body; promotes bone growth; needed to make cells and genetic material.	Green leafy vegetables; beans, nuts, fortified whole-grain cereals and breads, shellfish.
Manganese	Needed for healthy tendon and bone structure; component of several enzymes involved in metabolism.	Tea, coffee, bran, dried peas and beans, nuts.
Molybdenum	Component of enzymes essential for metabolism; helps regulate iron storage.	Dried peas and beans; dark green leafy vegetables; organ meats; whole-grain breads and cereals.
Phosphorus	Works with calcium to build and maintain bones and teeth; needed by certain enzymes to convert food into energy; promotes nerve and muscle function; helps maintain body's chemical balance.	Dairy products, egg yolks, meat, poultry, fish, legumes.
Potassium	Works with sodium to regulate fluid balance, promotes transmission of nerve impulses and proper muscle function, essential for metabolism.	Bananas, citrus fruits, dried fruits, deep yellow vegetables, potatoes, legumes, milk, bran cereal.
Selenium	Interacts with vitamin E to prevent breakdown of fats and body chemicals.	Poultry, seafood; egg yolks, whole-grain breads and cereals, mushrooms, onions, garlic.
Sodium	Helps maintain fluid balance.	Salt, processed foods, milk, water in some areas.
Sulfur	Needed to make hair and nails; component of several amino acids.	Wheat germ, dried peas and beans, beef, clams, peanuts.
Zinc	Needed in more than 100 enzymes instrumental in digestion and metabolism; essential for sexual maturation.	Beef, liver, oysters. yogurt, fortified cereals, wheat germ.

CARRY-ALONG FAST FOOD TABLES

Restaurant	Item	Calories	Calories from fat	Fat grams	% calories from fat
BURGER KING	**Burgers**				
	Whopper	630	342	38	54%
	Whopper with cheese	720	414	46	58%
	Double Whopper	920	531	59	58%
	Double Whopper with cheese	1010	567	63	56%
	Whopper Jr. Sandwich	400	216	24	54%
	Whopper Jr. with cheese	450	252	28	56%
	Big King Sandwich	640	378	42	59%
	Potato Salad	320	126	14	39%
	Mashed Potatoes with gravy	360	90	10	25%
	Bacon Cheeseburger	400	198	22	50%
	Double Cheeseburger	580	225	25	39%
	Bacon Double Cheeseburger	620	252	28	41%
	Sandwiches/Sides/Shakes				
	BK Big Fish Sandwich	720	387	43	54%
	BK Broiler Chicken Sandwich	530	90	10	17%
	Chicken Sandwich	710	234	26	33%
	Chicken Tenders	236	117	13	50%
	Chef Salad without dressing	178	81	9	46%
	Chunky Chicken Salad without dressing	142	36	4	25%
	Garden Salad without dressing	95	45	5	47%
	Dinner Salad without dressing	20	0	0	0%
	French Fries, small	250	117	13	47%
	Onion Rings	380	171	19	45%
	Chocolate Shake	440	90	10	20%
	Vanilla Shake	430	81	9	19%
DOMINO'S PIZZA	**Pizza**				
	12" Classic Hand-Tossed, 2 of 8 slices				
	Cheese	375	99	11	26%
	Pepperoni	448	162	18	35%
	Veggie	391	108	12	28%
	12" Thin Crust, 2 of 8 slices				
	Cheese	273	108	12	40%
	Pepperoni	347	162	18	47%
	Veggie	289	117	13	38%
	12" Deep Dish, 2 of 8 slices				
	Cheese	482	188	22	41%
	Pepperoni	647	298	32	45%
	Veggie	498	207	23	42%

Restaurant	Item	Calories	Calories from fat	Fat grams	% calories from fat
ARBY'S	**Sandwiches**				
	Arby's Melt 'n Cheese	340	187	15	55%
	Arby-Q	360	216	24	60%
	Beef 'n Cheddar	480	264	20	55%
	Junior Roast Beef	310	118	13	38%
	Regular Roast Beef	350	144	16	41%
	Super Roast Beef	470	207	23	44%
	Giant Roast Beef	480	206	23	43%
	French Dip	410	160	18	39%
	Hot Ham 'n Swiss	530	244	27	46%
	Italian	780	476	53	61%
	Philly Beef 'n Swiss	700	378	42	54%
	Roast Beef	760	433	48	57%
	Turkey	630	334	37	53%
	Chicken Bacon 'n Swiss	610	299	33	49%
	Chicken Breast Fillet	540	270	30	50%
	Chicken Cordon Bleu	630	315	35	50%
	Grilled Chicken Deluxe	450	198	22	44%
	Roast Chicken Club	520	250	28	48%
	Breakfast				
	Biscuit with Butter	280	154	17	55%
	Biscuit with Bacon	360	216	24	60%
	Biscuit with Ham	330	182	20	55%
	Biscuit with Sausage	460	299	33	65%
	Croissant (plain)	220	108	12	49%
	Croissant with Bacon	340	204	23	60%
	Croissant with Ham	310	180	20	58%
	Croissant with Sausage	440	286	32	65%
	French Toastix (no syrup)	370	152	17	41%
	Maple syrup	130	0	0	0%
	Light menu				
	Garden Salad	70	9	1	13%
	Grilled Chicken	280	45	5	16%
	Grilled Chicken Salad	210	40	4.5	19%
	Roast Chicken Deluxe	260	44	5	17%
	Roast Chicken Salad	160	22	2.5	14%
	Roast Turkey Deluxe	260	44	5	17%
	Side Salad	25	0	0	0%
	Sweets				
	Apple Turnover (iced)	420	143	16	34%
	Cheesecake (plain)	320	208	23	65%
	Cherry Turnover (iced)	410	144	16	35%
	Chocolate Chip Cookie	125	54	6	43%
	Chocolate Shake (14 oz.)	480	144	16	30%
	Other Flavor Shake (14 oz.)	470	136	15	29%

Restaurant	Item	Calories	Calories from fat	Fat grams	% calories from fat
KFC—Kentucky Fried Chicken	**Chicken**				
	Original Recipe Breast	400	216	24	54%
	Original Recipe Leg	140	81	9	58%
	Original Recipe Thigh	250	162	18	65%
	Extra Crispy Breast	470	252	28	54%
	Extra Crispy Leg	195	108	12	55%
	Extra Crispy Thigh	380	243	27	64%
	Sandwiches & other items				
	Hot Wings	471	297	33	63%
	Crispy Strips	300	144	16	48%
	Original Recipe Chicken Sandwich with sauce	450	198	22	44%
	Original Recipe Chicken Sandwich without sauce	360	117	13	33%
	Honey BBQ Flavored Chicken Sandwich without sauce	310	54	6	17%
	Sides				
	BBQ Baked Beans	190	27	3	14%
	Biscuit	180	90	10	50%
	Cole Slaw	232	126	14	54%
	Corn on the Cob	150	18	2	12%
	Potato Salad	230	126	14	55%
	Mashed Potatoes with gravy	120	54	6	45%
TACO BELL	**Burritos**				
	Bean Burrito	370	110	12	30%
	7-Layer Burrito	520	198	22	38%
	Burrito Supreme—Beef	520	200	22	38%
	Burrito Supreme—Chicken	430	170	18	40%
	Grilled Stuft Burrito—Beef	410	140	16	34%
	Various items				
	Gordita Supreme—Chicken	300	120	14	40%
	Zesty Chicken Border Bowl without dressing	460	170	19	37%
	Tostada	250	110	12	44%
	Mexican Pizza	540	310	35	57%
	Tacos				
	Taco	210	110	12	52%
	Taco Supreme	260	140	16	54%
	Soft Taco—Beef	210	90	10	43%
	Soft Taco—Chicken	190	60	7	32%
	Other items				
	Cheese Quesadilla	490	250	28	51%
	Nachos	320	260	18	81%
	Nachos Supreme	440	210	24	48%
	Chalupa Supreme—Beef	380	200	23	53%
	Chalupa Supreme—Chicken	360	180	20	50%

Restaurant	Item	Calories	Calories from fat	Fat grams	% calories from fat
McDONALD'S	**Sandwiches**				
	Hamburger	270	81	9	30%
	Cheeseburger	320	117	13	37%
	Quarter Pounder	430	189	21	44%
	Quarter Pounder with cheese	530	270	30	51%
	Big Mac	570	288	32	51%
	Filet-O-Fish	470	234	26	50%
	Grilled Chicken Deluxe	440	180	20	41%
	Grilled Chicken Deluxe without mayo	300	45	5	15%
	Sides & McNuggets				
	Chicken McNuggets, 4 pieces	190	99	11	52%
	Chicken McNuggets, 6 pieces	290	153	17	53%
	Barbeque Sauce, 1 package	45	0	0	0%
	French Fries, small	210	90	10	43%
	Garden Salad	35	0	0	0%
	Grilled Chicken Salad Deluxe	120	14	1.5	11%
	Ranch Dressing, 2-oz. packet	230	189	21	82%
	Fat Free Herb Vinaigrette	50	0	0	0%
	Breakfast items				
	Egg McMuffin	290	108	12	37%
	Bacon, Egg & Cheese Biscuit	540	306	34	57%
	Hash Browns	130	72	8	55%
	Hot Cakes (plain)	340	72	8	21%
	Breakfast Burrito	320	180	20	56%
	Low Fat Apple Bran Muffin	300	27	3	9%
	Cheese Danish	400	189	21	47%
	Sweets				
	Vanilla Cone (red. fat)	150	41	4.5	27%
	Hot Fudge Sundae	340	108	12	32%
	McDonaldland Cookies	180	45	5	25%
	Vanilla Shake, small	360	81	9	23%
SUBWAY	**Sandwiches**				
	6" Veggie Delite	232	27	3	12%
	6" Classic Italian B.M.T.	450	189	21	42%
	6" Cold Cut Trio	374	126	14	34%
	6" Ham	293	45	5	15%
	6" Roast Beef	296	45	5	15%
	6" Subway Seafood & Crab	338	81	9	24%
	6" Subway Club	304	45	5	15%
	6" Turkey	282	36	4	13%
	6" Tuna with light mayo	378	126	14	33%
	6" Meatball	413	135	15	33%

Organizations That Can Help

These organizations can help you find aid for mental health issues. If you do not have Internet access at home, public libraries have computers with Internet service that you can use for free.

American Academy of Child and Adolescent Psychiatry (www.aacap.org) provides information to help understand and treat childhood developmental, behavioral, and mental disorders.

American Association of Marriage and Family Therapy (www.aamft.org) will help you locate a family therapist in your area, as well as find books, articles, and information on family problems and how to address them.

Boys and Girls Clubs of America (www.bgca.org/) will help kids find recreation and companionship opportunities away from home with adult care and supervision.

Center for Fathers, Families, and Workforce Development Headquarters (www.cfwd.org) will provide assistance and support in many areas, including parenting skills, life skills, child support, health and mental health issues, youth services, and referral services.

The Depressed Child (www.aacap.org/publications/factsfam/depressd.htm) provides a fact sheet that presents parents with an overview of childhood and adolescent depression, including signs and symptoms, diagnosis, and appropriate treatment.

Federation of Families for Children's Mental Health (www.ffcmh.org) is a national parent-run advocacy and support organization for children and their families aimed at helping youths with emotional, behavioral, or mental disorders.

Kids and Eating Disorders (www.kidshealth.org/kid/health_problems/learning_problem/eatdisorder.html) is for use by kids and provides information on body image and eating disorders.

National Fatherhood Initiative (www.fatherhood.org) encourages fathers to take a positive, active role in their children's lives.

National Indian Child Welfare Association (www.nicwa.org) is a national group dedicated to the well-being of American Indian children and families.

National Dissemination Center for Children with Disabilities (www.nichcy.org) provides information on disabilities and disability-related issues, with a special focus on children and youths through age 22.

National Latino Children's Institute (www.nlci.org) focuses exclusively on children, working in public education, healthy communities, and helping children express themselves.

National Mental Health and Education Center (www.naspcenter.org/ index2.html) provides information in English and Spanish about mental health education for teachers and parents.

National Network for Youth (www.nn4youth.org) includes more than 800 organizations advocating for young people who have been challenged by abuse, neglect, family conflict, shortage of resources, prejudice, and other challenges.

Research & Training Center for Children's Mental Health (http://rtckids.fmhi.nsf.edu) lists services for children and adolescents with serious emotional disabilities.

Research & Training Center on Family Support and Children's Mental Health (www.rtc.pdx.edu/) tells you how to find effective community-based family-centered services for families and their children who may be affected by mental, emotional or behavioral disorders.

Soy Unica! Soy Latina! (www.soyunica.gov) is a public education campaign to help Hispanic girls and their mothers build and enhance self-esteem, mental health, decision-making, and assertiveness skills.

Stepfamily Association of America (www.saafamilies.org) is a nonprofit organization dedicated to harmonious stepfamily relationships.

The Sweeney Alliance (www.sweeneyalliance.org) is a nationally recognized nonprofit organization that provides help to families and professionals coping with grief and stress, teaching children and adults how to reinvest in life and living following a life-altering event such as the death of a loved one, divorce, violence, neglect, or disability.

United Parents (www.unitedparents.org) offers support, assistance, education, and resources for families of children with emotional, behavior, and mental disorders.

VERB (www.VERBparents.com, www.VERBnow.com) is a program sponsored by the Centers for Disease Control (CDC) to combat childhood obesity by promoting healthier lifestyles and physical activity among youths aged 9 to 13, with the support of parents and other partners in the community.

Sources

AACE Power of Prevention. Automated BMI Calculator (www.powerofprevention.com).

Allison, D. B., K. R. Fontaine, and J. E. Manson. "Annual Deaths Attributable to Obesity in the United States." *Journal of the American Medical Association* 282 (1999): 1530–8.

Anderson, Kristin J., and Donna Cavallaro. "Parents or Pop Culture? Children's Heroes and Role Models." *Childhood Education* 78, no. 3 (Spring 2002): Research Library, 161–8.

Bar-or, Oded. "Health Benefits of Physical Activity During Childhood and Adolescence." *President's Council on Physical Fitness and Sports Research Digest,* ser. 2, no. 4 (December 1995).

Beans, Bruce. "Stretching Your Way to Success." *Starting Out Healthy* (Spring 2003). Moorestown, New Jersey: Health Ink and Vitality Communications (http://12.31.13.115/healthyliving/fitness/mar03fitnessstretchsuccess.htm).

Bjorntorp, Per, and B. N. Brodoff. *Obesity.* Philadelphia: J. B. Lippincott, 1992.

Critser, Greg. *Fat Land.* New York: Houghton Mifflin, 2003.

Dallman, M. F., N. Pecoraro, S. F. Akana, S. E. La Fleur, F. Gomez, H. Houshyar, M. E. Bell, S. Bhatnagar, K. D. Laugero, and S. Manalo. "Chronic Stress and Obesity: A New View of 'Comfort Food.'" *Proceedings of the National Academy of Sciences U.S.A.* 100, no. 20 (September 30, 2003): 11696–701. Epub September 15, 2003.

Dwyer, T., J. F. Sallis, L. Blizzard, R. Lazarus, and K. Dean. "Relation of Academic Performance to Physical Activity and Fitness in Children." *Pediatric Exercise Science* 13 (2001): 225–38.

Eisenberg, Marla E., Dianne Neumark-Sztainer, and Mary Story. "Associations of Weight-Based Teasing and Emotional Well-Being among Adolescents." *Archives of Pediatrics and Adolescent Medicine* 157 (August 2003): 733–8.

Epstein, Leonard. "Childhood Obesity." *Pediatric Clinics of North America* (1985): 364.

Epstein, Leonard. "Effects of Diet Plus Exercise on Weight Change in Parents and Children." *Journal of Consulting Clinical Psychology* 52 (1984): 429–37.

Flegal, K. M., and R. P. Troiano. "Changes in the Distribution of Body Mass Index of Adults and Children in the U.S. Population." *International Journal of Obesity and Related Metabolic Disorders* 24 (2000): 807–18.

Earl Ford. "Insulin Resistance Syndrome: The Public Health Challenge." *Endocrine Practice* 9, Supplement 2 (2003): 23–26.

M. W. Gillman, S. L. Rifas-Sherman, A. L. Frazier, H. R. Rockett, C. A. Camargo, A. E. Field, C. S. Berkey, and G. A. Colditz. "Family Dinner and Diet Quality among Older Children and Adolescents." *Archives of Family Medicine* 9 (2000): 235–40.

Gortmaker, S. L., W. H. Dietz, and L. W. Y. Cheung. "Inactivity, Diet and the Fattening of America." *Journal of the American Dietetic Association* 90 (1990): 1247–52.

Gortmaker, S. L., A. Must, A. M. Sobol, K. Peterson, G. A. Colditz, and W. H. Dietz. "Television Viewing as a Cause of Increasing Obesity among Children in the United States, 1986–1990." *Archives of Pediatrics and Adolescent Medicine* 150 (1996): 356–62

Harnack, L., J. Stang, and M. Story. "Soft Drink Consumption among U.S. School Children and Adolescents: Nutritional Consequences." *Journal of the American Dietetic Association* 99 (April 1999): 436–41.

Iwane, M., M. Arita, S. Tomimoto, O. Satani, M. Matsumoto, and I. Miyashita Nishio. "Walking 10,000 Steps/Day or More Reduces Blood Pressure and Sympathetic Nervous Activity in Mild Essential Hypertension." *Hypertension Research* 23 (November 2000): 573–80.

Jacobson, Michael, and Bruce Maxwell. *What Are We Feeding Our Kids?* New York: Workman Press, 1994.

Keays J. J., and K. R. Allison. *Canadian Journal of Public Health* 86, no. 1 (January–February 1995): 62–65.

Lin, B. H., J. Guthrie, and E. Frazao. "Nutrient Contributions of Food Away from Home." In "Eating Habits: Changes and Consequences," edited by E. Frazao. *Agriculture Information Bulletin* 750 (1999): 213. Washington, D.C.: USDA.

Ludwig, D. S., J. A. Majzoub, A. Al-Zahrani, G. E. Dallal, I. Blanco, and S. B. Roberts. "High Glycemic Index Foods, Overeating, and Obesity." *Pediatrics* 103, no. 3 (March 1999): e26.

Luepker, R. V. "How Physically Active Are American Children and What Can We Do about It?" *International Journal of Obesity and Related Metabolic Disorders.* Supplement 2 (March 1999): S12–17.

National Association for Sport and Physical Education. *Shape of the Nation Report.* 2001 (www.aahperd.org/naspe/pdf_files/shape_nation.pdf).

Natow, Annette B., and Jo-Ann Heslin. *The Most Complete Food Counter.* New York: Pocket Books, 1999.

Nestle, Marion. *Food Politics: How the Food Industry Influences Nutrition and Health.* Berkeley and Los Angeles: University of California Press, 2003.

Pate, Russell, Chuck Corbin, and Bob Pangrazi. "Physical Activity for Young People." *President's Council on Physical Fitness and Sports Research Digest,* ser. 3, no. 3 (September 1998).

Pereira, M. A., D. R. Jacobs Jr., J. J. Pins, S. K. Raatz, M. D. Gross, J. L. Slavin, and E. R. Seaquist. "Effect of Whole Grains on Insulin Sensitivity in Overweight Hyperinsulinemic Adults." *American Journal of Clinical Nutrition* 75 (May 2002): 848–55.

Piscatella, Jo. "How to Fatproof Your Child." *Mastercard Dining Out Survey,* 1997.

President's Council on Physical Fitness and Sports. *Get Fit! A Handbook for Youth Ages 6–17: How to Get in Shape to Meet the President's Challenge.* Washington, D.C., 2001 (www.fitness.gov/getfit.pdf).

Rolls, Barbara J., Diane Engell, and Leann Birch. "Serving Portions Size Influences Five-Year-Old but Not Three-Year-Old Children's Food Intakes." *Journal of the American Dietetic Association* 100 (February 2000): 232–4.

SOURCES

Satter, Ellyn. *How to Get Your Kid to Eat . . . But Not Too Much.* Palo Alto, Calif.: Bull Publishing, 1993.

Schlosser, Eric. *Fast Food Nation.* Boston: Houghton-Mifflin, 2001.

Schwimmer, J. B., T. M. Burwinkle, and J. W. Varni. "Health-Related Quality of Life of Severely Obese Children and Adolescents." *Journal of the American Medical Association* 289, no. 14 (Apr. 9, 2003): 1813–9.

State of Idaho Department of Education. "Start Today for a Healthy Tomorrow." Adapted from the American Dietetic Association/Foundation and Kellogg Company (www.sde.state.id.us/child/docs/tips.pdf).

Stunkard, A. J., T. I. Sorenson, C. Hanis, T. W. Teasdale, R. Chakraborty, W. J. Schull, and F. Schulsinger. "An Adoption Study of Human Obesity." *New England Journal of Medicine* 314 (1986): 193–8.

Taylor, W. C., A. K. Yancey, J. Leslie, N. G. Murray, S. S. Cummings, S. A. Sharkey, C. Wert, J. James, O. Miles, and W. J. McCarthy. "Physical Activity among African American and Latino Middle School Girls: Consistent Beliefs, Expectations, and Experiences across Two Sites." *Women and Health* 30, no. 2 (1999): 67–82.

Troiano, R. P., K. M. Flegal, and R. J. Kuczmarski. "Overweight Prevalence and Trends for Children and Adolescents." *Archives of Pediatric and Adolescent Medicine* 149 (1995): 1085–91.

U.S. Department of Agriculture, Agricultural Research Service. *USDA National Nutrient Database for Standard Reference,* Release 15 (2002). Nutrient Data Laboratory Home Page (www.nal.usda.gov/fnic/foodcomp).

U.S. Department of Health and Human Services. "National Children and Youth Fitness Study." *Journal of Physical Education, Recreation, and Dance* 56 (1985): 44–90.

U. S. Department of Health and Human Services. *The Surgeon General's Call to Action to Prevent and Decrease Overweight and Obesity* (http://bookstore.gpo.gov/), stock no. 017-001-00551-7.

Van Amelsvoort, J. M., A. van der Beek, and J. J. Stam. "Dietary Influence on the Insulin Function in the Epididymal Fat Cell of the Wistar Rat." *Annals of Nutrition and Metabolism* 32 (1988): 138–48.

Williams, C. L., L. L. Hayman, S. R. Daniels, T. N. Robinson, J. Steinberger, S. Paridon, and T. Bazzarre. "Cardiovascular Health in Childhood: A Statement for Health Professionals from the Committee on Atherosclerosis, Hypertension, and Obesity in the Young (AHOY) of the Council on Cardiovascular Disease in the Young, American Heart Association." *Circulation* 106, no. 9 (Aug. 27, 2002): 1178.

Winter, Greg. "Some States Fight Junk Food Sales in Schools." *New York Times,* September 9, 2001.

Zive, M. M., G. C. Frank-Spohrer, J. F. Sallis, T. L. McKenzie, J. P. Elder, C. C. Berry, S. L. Broyles, and P. R. Nader. "Determinants of Dietary Intake in a Sample of White and Mexican-American Children." *Journal of the American Dietetic Association* 98, no. 11 (1998): 1282–9.

Index

O'Shea, Michael, 163
Overeating
    early puberty and, 45
    myth of instinct against,
        32–34
    as symptom of something
        deeper, 21
Overweight
    medical risks of, 17–18
    nothing funny about, 5
    number one health problem
        in America, 2
    statistics, 9, 28
    varied causes of, 24

P
Palm oil, 9
Pancreas, 19
Parents
    can change lazy habits,
        114
    children's eating habits and,
        21
    children's self-esteem and,
        86
    and denial about child's
        weight, 1
    disagreements between, 15
    improvements to health of,
        4
    as motivators, 72
    as role models, 28, 72
    as supporters of active chil-
        dren, 124
    as workshop participants,
        14
P.E.4Life, Web site, 208
Pediatricians, see Physicians
Pedometer, 122
Percent daily values, part of
    food label, 92
Perry, William "Refrigerator,"
    17
Personal meal plan, 104–106
Phen-fen, 13
Photocopy materials, 213–248
Physical activity, see Activity,
    physical
Physical education
    children and, 12

programs to restore in
    schools, 208
statistics, 15
Physical fitness test, inability
    to pass, statistics, 16
Physicians
    best resource for informa-
        tion, 37
    questions for, 37–38
    weight charts and, 30
Points-reward system, 43, 53,
    73, 87, 111
Popular culture, influence of,
    36–37
Portion sizes, 9, 81–82
Prader-Willi syndrome, 11
President's Council on
    Physical Fitness and
    Sports
    Challenge test, 48–52, 166,
        209–210
    recommendations of, 161
    research digests, 208
Protein foods, 64
    single servings of, 100–101
Puberty
    early, 45
    obesity and, 52
Pull-ups, 51
Push-away (exercise), 166
Push-ups, 50
Pyramid, see Activity pyramid;
    Food guide pyramid
PYY, potential treatment for
    obesity, 11

Q
Questions
    about buddy system, 78, 80
    about changes, 152
    about exercise, 115
    about food choices, 121
    about food servings, 102
    about holiday foods, 144
    about menu planning, 106,
        107
    about physical activities, 84
    about restaurants, 132
    to ask doctor, 37–38
    during role-play, 142–143

for parents, 80–81
for personal journal, 70–71,
    85–86, 108, 123, 135–136,
    145, 157

R
Read-aloud, see Food for
    Thought
Recipes, 177–204
    appetizers, 178–180
    breads, 180–183
    desserts, 197–202
    drinks, 202–204
    entrées, 189–197
    salads, 186–188
    vegetables, 183–185
Recreation areas, need to
    increase, 210
Reduced fat, defined, 94
Relaxation, breathing and,
    173
Restaurant Tips (table), 131
Restaurants
    Carry-Along Fast Food
        Tables (reproducible),
        247–248
    eating out at, 125–136
    ethnic, 133
    fast-food, 128
    limiting time in, 109
    tips (table), 131
Reward system, 15, 53
    devising, 43–44
Rice, Stephen, 176
Role models, parents as, 28
Role-playing, 130
    difficult scenarios, 153–155
    special occasions, 141–142
Ruth, Babe, 17

S
Saccharin, 97–98
Salads
    Caesar Salad, 186
    Hometown Salad, 188
    Japanese-Style Cucumbers,
        186
    June's Salad, 188
    Nana Sheila's Fruit Salad,
        187

About the Author

Naomi Neufeld, MD, FACE, is a nationally recognized authority on childhood weight problems. A graduate of Brown University who received her medical degree from Tufts University School of Medicine, Dr. Neufeld has been working with overweight children and their families for more than 25 years.

She is the founder and medical director of KidShape, the groundbreaking weight-loss program that has helped thousands of children and their families lose weight and get on the road to a lifetime of healthy eating and activity since it was founded in 1986.

She is regarded as the "go-to" expert on childhood weight problems, and as a strong advocate of family involvement. She is regularly quoted both in print media and on television. Her family-centered approach has been featured on *Oprah, Eye on America, The Today Show*, and *Discovery*, as well as in *Time, Newsweek,* and *Family Circle* magazines, among many others.

Dr. Neufeld is well known and widely respected in her field. She is an attending physician and former director of pediatric endocrinology at Cedars-Sinai Medical Center and Clinical Professor of Pediatrics at the UCLA School of Medicine. She is the author of the chapter on childhood obesity in *The Atlas of Clinical Endocrinology,* as well as more than 60 research and review articles and abstracts on pediatric endocrinology and obesity. She is a Charter Member of the American Association of Clinical Endocrinologists and serves on its board of directors. She was elected a Fellow of the American College of Endocrinology in 2002, and is a member of several other professional organizations, including the Lawson Wilkins Pediatric Endocrine Society, the Society for Pediatric Research, the American Diabetes Association, and the Juvenile Diabetes Foundation.

Dr. Neufeld is deeply involved in research into the causes and cures for child and adolescent obesity, and has been in the vanguard in identifying, studying, and reporting on these issues. In 1992, she received a pilot grant from the National Institutes of Health (NIH) to define type 2 diabetes in minority youth, and presented her data at the 1994 American Diabetes Association meeting, four years before other researchers began reporting similar findings. In another NIH-funded study, she did innovative work establishing that excess weight gain and obesity are perpetuated by impaired utilization of calories for heat in newborns of diabetic mothers.

She is a recipient of the Clinical Investigation Award from the National Institute of Arthritis, Diabetes, and Digestive and Kidney Disorders (part of NIH) and has served on the Ad Hoc Consensus Committee on Type 2 Diabetes in Children of the American Diabetes Association.

She has received more than a dozen research grants from such funding sources as the Juvenile Diabetes Foundation, the American Lung Association, and the March of Dimes–Birth Defects Foundation. Her current research is funded through grants from the Josephine Gumbiner Foundation, the Wellpoint Foundation, the California Nutrition Network, the California Department of Health (Division of Cancer Prevention), and the Children and Families Commission of Orange County (California). Her clinical research on medical problems associated with childhood obesity has been supported by grants from Bristol-Myers Squibb, Novo-Nordisk, Elli Lilly Foundation, and Pharmacia Corporation. The Children and Families First Commission of Ventura County (California) is funding the ongoing development and pilot testing of the KinderShape curriculum, a new early intervention program modeled after KidShape.